KV-033-520

faking it!

faking it!

how to look like a natural-born beauty

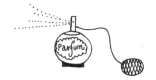

Sarah Barclay

CARLTON

For my grandmother MBS

The average girl would rather have beauty than brains
because she knows the average man can see
much better than he can think

Anonymous, quoted in *Ladies Home Journal*, 1947

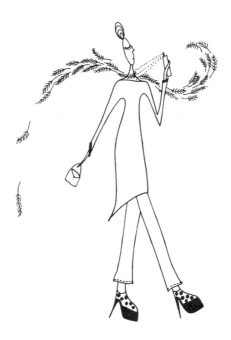

THIS IS A CARLTON BOOK

Text copyright ©1999 Sarah Barclay
Design and illustrations copyright © 1999 Carlton Books Limited

This edition published by Carlton Books Limited 1999
20 St Anne's Court
Wardour Street
London W1V 3AW

This book is sold subject to the condition that it shall not, by way of trade or otherwise, be lent, resold, hired out or otherwise circulated without the publisher's prior written consent in any form of cover or binding other than that in which it is published and without a similar condition including this condition being imposed upon the subsequent purchaser.

All rights reserved.

A CIP catalogue for this book is available from the British Library.

ISBN 1 85868 680 6

Printed and bound in Great Britain.

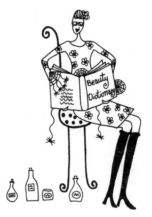

Senior executive editor: Venetia Penfold
Copy editor: Lisa Dyer
Project editor: Zia Mattocks
Art director: Penny Stock
Senior art editor: Barbara Zuñiga
Illustrations: Carol Morley
Production: Garry Lewis

contents

introduction

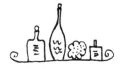

It has always been a mystery to me that for such a light-hearted, self-indulgent subject as beauty, books written on the topic are more serious than a DIY enthusiast's tool box. They either promise impossibly unlikely results, not to mention endless exercises demonstrated by models in terrible sportswear, or they assume you take make-up so seriously that a special PHD in the subject should follow swiftly after working your way through the text. By the time you have done, digested, applied and removed everything you are told to use, there is little room for doing anything else, let alone to have fun.

But it is confusing. The beauty industry is a billion-dollar machine selling every conceivable lotion and potion for every real and imaginary beauty problem or fashion. Some are so deliciously packaged that it is hard not to be seduced by their superficial charms, while others are like talented physics students – rather unglamorous-looking but produce brilliant results. For most of us, knowing what to buy and apply is one holy grail, dealing with real-life situations is another.

Feminists may despair that we are not wobbling our thighs with pride or rejecting bank-balance draining cosmetics in favour of more important things in life (like buying their bossy books), but I think they have missed the point. If you believe you look good, you will feel better and the world seems a nicer place.

Faking It! is all about cheating the system. It is about looking ravishing at all times without looking like you have tried for a moment. So, whether you are slinking around in a bikini on a summer holiday or dealing with an action-packed hearty weekend, there is no reason why anyone should be left in any doubt about your heavenly, natural beauty.

chapter one

the summer holiday

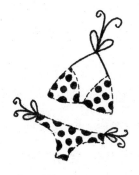

There is something rather cruel about summer holidays. All year long we are bombarded with advertisements showing perfectly toned women and strong-jawed men snogging under palm trees or frolicking, hysterical with laughter, in turquoise sea. Then off we go, cellulite-coated thighs wobbling, bikini lines overflowing, and wonder why we feel a little self-conscious.

And the agony is not just confined to a beach holiday. Just as destinations have become more varied, so too have the holiday beauty nightmares. Our mothers may have breathed a little sigh of despair when they watched Ursula Andress wade alluringly out of the sea in *Dr No* in the 1960s, but we have the added inspiration – or torture – of ravishing heroines in action movies surviving in equatorial rainforests without so much as a hairy armpit or an unplucked eyebrow.

If you are feeling at all unconfident about your appearance, preparing for a summer holiday of any description makes matters worse. Whether you are trying on a bikini in a changing room with lighting that makes you look like a fluorescent Sumo wrestler or you arrive at your destination only to find an array of cellulite-free sirens slinking around the pool, confidence-building 'faking it' tactics need to be employed at every opportunity.

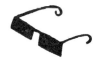

countdown to fitness

Most of us have found ourselves attempting stomach-flattening sit-ups the night before a summer holiday. The consoling thought is that by the time most women have developed a noticeable helping of cellulite, men, after years of pouring pints of lager down their throats, are beginning to get paunches and go bald. The great advantage women have is that they can swathe their limbs in sarongs and slip discreetly into a pool. Men just seem to wear smaller and tighter swimming trunks. The good news is that we all feel more perky during the spring and summer months, so take advantage of this increased energy and start exercising. To be of any real health benefit and to notice significant improvement in muscle tone, an exercise programme should begin at least two to three months before the holiday.

If you want to tone up but loathe all the body-beautiful types in gyms and cannot afford, or admit to having, a personal fitness trainer, try yoga. Yoga lengthens and tones muscles, making you look leaner, and although the exercises increase strength, you will not build muscle and turn into a female gorilla. Because deep breathing is fundamental to yoga, you will feel more relaxed after doing the exercises – an added benefit when it comes to the trauma of shopping for swimwear. Practise yogic breathing throughout the posture exercises.

yogic breathing

Your breathing should be deep and should be from the stomach, rather than from the chest.

1. Lie on the floor with your legs stretched out and your arms at your sides with your palms facing up.

2. Draw breath in through the nose, down the throat and out again through the nose. This should make a slight whispering or snoring sound. As you inhale, your stomach should swell; as you exhale, it should deflate.

3. Repeat several times before moving on to the postures.

posture 1

This easy exercise tones the arms, legs, stomach and bottom. Do it first thing in the morning to help you wake up.

1. Sit on the floor with your back straight and your legs outstretched. Your hands should rest on the floor, palms down, with your elbows bent at the sides of your body.

2. Using your arms and buttock muscles, push your body up off the floor until your arms are completely straight. Your legs should be straight with your feet flat on the floor.

3. With your body still raised off the floor, push your pelvis up as high as possible and hold the position for four deep breaths.

4. Repeat four times.

posture 2

A toner for the legs, back, arms and bottom, this posture is a good follow-up to the above exercise.

1. Kneel on the floor with your arms straight and your palms flat on the floor. Make sure your back is straight and your weight is evenly distributed.

2. Flex your feet in, against the floor, so your toes are pressing down on the floor.

3. Push your bottom up in the air, keeping your arms straight, until your legs are completely straight. Your heels will automatically come off the ground.

4. Press your heels down gently, keeping your bottom as high as you can and feeling your legs lengthening. Your head should hang down comfortably. Hold for four breaths.

5. Repeat four times.

cellulite busting

If you are determined to do something about 'orange peel' thighs, start an anti-cellulite programme about two months before the holiday. I am not talking about just rubbing some expensive anti-cellulite cream into your thighs every day and expecting a miracle. I do not know a single beauty editor who wholeheartedly believes that any of the brands on the market really have a pronounced effect; some do absolutely nothing except make you poorer. However, combining regular massage using ingredients that stimulate the skin and the circulation (many of which are found in these creams) with the right diet and regular exercise does seem to improve the appearance of cellulite, and in some cases removes it altogether.

Although cellulite is not medically recognized in the UK, anyone who suffers from it knows what it looks like. Cellulite has nothing to do with being overweight; some of the slimmest, youngest models have it. It tends to develop at times of hormonal change, such as puberty, going on the Pill, pregnancy and menopause, and varies in severity. Other possible culprits are poor circulation, a lack of exercise and a poor diet, which leads to overloading the body with toxins that lodge themselves in fat cells. Stress has also been cited as a cause, but is often accompanied by excessive consumption of stimulants, such as coffee, alcohol and nicotine, which are known toxins.

A few years ago the bumpy fat deposits were blamed on poor circulation and the treatment involved breaking down the fat using rubbery massage tools and a special cream. However, this sort of aggressive massage was deemed damaging to the skin and, if anything, had the potential to make cellulite look worse. Rather than promising to melt away the fat, some of the latest anti-cellulite creams claim to firm and tone the skin that surrounds cellulite (rather like strengthening a rubber coating) so that the cellulite is less visible, and phrases like 'body contouring and sculpting' entered the marketing vocabulary. Massaging thighs with a cream, gel or oil will make skin look smoother and improve local circulation. Bear in mind that halfway through a cellulite-shifting programme, whether in a salon or at home, cellulite may seem to get worse (as the fat cells break down) before it improves, but quite quickly your body and regular massage will disperse the dislodged 'waste matter'.

salon treatments

Spa or beauty salon anti-cellulite programmes are probably the most effective treatments. However, these are expensive and are only worth doing if you are prepared to pay for a number of sessions. Different salons offer a variety of approaches, ranging from aromatherapy to high-tech microcurrent massage. The method you choose largely depends on personal preference – some are messier and more claustrophobic than others. Although the treatments vary, the aim is identical: to increase the body's circulation and, in doing so, speed up the elimination of toxins. Many anti-cellulite programmes combine a number of the treatments listed below:

Aromatherapy Often combined with body brushing (see pages 20–1), an aromatherapy treatment involves massage with detoxifying essential oils. Because essential oils sink into the skin and enter the bloodstream (which is why they are potentially risky if used on pregnant women), the system is deeply stimulated.

Lymphatic drainage massage The lymphatic system is your body's toxin-clearing mechanism. It is an intricate network of minute tubes that help disperse harmful bacteria and toxins. When the system becomes sluggish, toxins remain trapped in the body, theoretically contributing to cellulite build-up. Lymphatic drainage massage speeds up the natural waste-disposal process. A clear indication of a good lymphatic massage is increased passing of urine for several hours following the treatment.

Thalassotherapy Any type of therapy that uses marine extracts, particularly seaweed, is known as thalassotherapy. Anti-cellulite treatments commonly include a sea salt rub-down, which works the same way as body brushing for an aromatherapy treatment. The body is then smothered in warm, pulverized seaweed or marine mud to aid detoxification. The process usually involves being wrapped in a plastic sheet and left to sweat for about 20 minutes. If you do not like the aroma of seaweed or the smell of mud, this treatment is not for you.

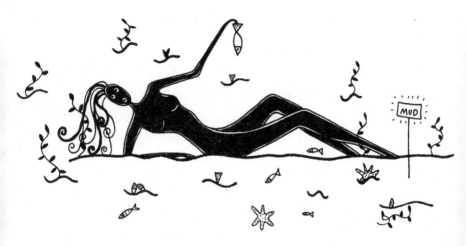

Microcurrents Galvanic currents or microcurrents work on the same body-stimulating principle as the other treatments. Electrodes or rods conducting a mild current are attached to the skin. With the circulation stimulated, the lymphatic system operates more efficiently to dispel waste matter from the body.

home treatments

One of the most effective changes you can make towards banishing cellulite from your body for good is dietary, and it is not nearly as hard as it sounds. For the most successful results, combine several – or all – of the following cellulite-beating strategies:

Diet changes Cutting out, or at least down on, caffeine and alcohol will help give your body's natural cleansing system more energy to dispel toxin-loaded cellulite. If you smoke, give up. Not only does it make the body more tired, so less able to rid itself of toxins, but smoking also destroys the body's reserves of vitamin C, an important skin and circulation supporter.

Reduce your intake of wheat and dairy foods. Wheat makes the body sluggish and can cause bloating and fluid retention. Dairy products contain large helpings of fat and congest the body. Although eliminating foods containing either or both of these substances entirely is almost impossible and nutritionally risky, after a few weeks of cutting down on them you should notice an increase in your energy levels, an indication that your toxin-elimination system is functioning more efficiently. (See also the detox diet, page 127.)

Water Replacing endless cups of caffeine-laden coffee, tea and carbonated sugary drinks with mineral water is probably the most important part of an anti-cellulite campaign. If you do not do this, you cannot 'flush' the body out and fully cleanse the system. Also, you will merely

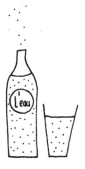

replace all the toxins you have enthusiastically body brushed and massaged away with a large helping of new ones. Drinking one to two litres of water a day is a positive, if not good, start. If your urine is anything but the palest yellow, you should be drinking more water. Apart from improving your skin, you will also have more energy and sleep better. Opt for still rather than sparkling mineral water to prevent unnecessary bloating.

Body brushing This stimulates the skin and improves circulation, which jump-starts the body into eliminating waste. In addition to improving circulation, your skin will feel softer and look brighter too, since the brushing action has an exfoliating effect, sloughing away the dull-looking surface layer of dead skin cells. Body brushes can be found in high street beauty shops, department stores and chemists and cost about the same as a box of Belgian chocolates. Begin by gently brushing on dry skin in one direction only, from the soles of the feet up along the legs to the buttocks. Brush from the hands along the arms to the shoulders and chest. All strokes should move towards the heart. When you brush, use a firm but gentle pressure. The idea is to brush away dead skin cells and stimulate the skin, not to damage it. At first you may find body brushing a little uncomfortable, even quite rough, but after a few days you will be able to increase the pressure. The best time to brush is first thing in the morning before a shower.

Massage After a bath or shower, firmly massage cellulite areas with an oil, cream or gel. Olive oil or an ordinary body cream can be used if you are feeling thrifty and disdainful of swanky products. Massage will aid the dispersal of toxins, stimulate sluggish fat cells and help work any detoxifying ingredients in the cream into the skin. Always massage in circular motions with firm pressure, working up the body towards the heart.

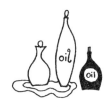

anti-cellulite checklist

- ❤ DO body brush.
- ❤ DO massage the skin.
- ❤ DO drink plenty of still water.
- ❤ DO cut down on your consumption of dairy foods, wheat, alcohol and caffeine.
- ❤ DO exercise, even if it is just walking more and faster.
- ❤ DON'T smoke.
- ❤ DON'T expect results for at least three weeks.
- ❤ DON'T take cellulite too seriously. Instead, comfort yourself that toxic build-up is just a sign of a life of pleasure and hedonism.

sun protection

Two weeks before your holiday is the time to invest in sun protection cream. This may sound a bit premature and not in the jolly spirit of going on a pre-holiday shop, but they cost far more than you think and you will use far more than you imagine. Of course we all want to guard against skin cancer but preventing ageing is also a serious beauty necessity. Damage caused by ultraviolet rays is responsible for 80 per cent of fine lines and wrinkles. Thanks to decades of sun-drenched summer holidays and the fashion for having a deep tan, skin cancer is now on the increase in the UK. Do not be tempted by low factors or oils. They will offer minimal protection and will simply fry your skin. The skin will turn red and peel a few days later anyway, and your tan will not last. Unless you want to end up looking like a prune, avoid sunbeds like the plague. They do nothing for the health of the skin and just make it age faster.

UVA and UVB filters Sun protection factors (SPFs) do not protect against ageing, but only against the burning rays of UVB, which can ultimately cause damaged, aged skin, and skin cancer. UVA filters protect against UVA rays, which reach into the depths of the skin's structure and damage fibres that give skin its firmness and wrinkle-free appearance. You need a sunscreen that protects from both UVA and UVB; think of the SPF as your healthy skin filter and the UVA screen as your long-term beauty investment.

Buy an SPF15 that also includes a maximum UVA filter in the formula (the level of screening against UVA is represented by stars on the packaging). You should have one cream for the face and another formula for the body, both SPF15. This is the minimum amount of protection dermatologists recommend.

Chemical and physical blocks Chemical sunscreens sink into the skin and protect it from within by absorbing ultraviolet rays. Physical sunscreens (such as titanium dioxide) sit on the skin's surface and reflect light away, like tiny mirrors. Some of the best sunscreens contain both elements. Do not be confused or seduced by confident claims of such-and-such '-free' screens. Some chemical sunscreens are perfectly effective and well tolerated by the skin, whereas others can be irritating. However, if you have sensitive skin, choose a physical block.

Antioxidants and added ingredients Research has shown that antioxidants not only protect against damage from the sun, but actually help reverse the effects of previous damage a little, so it is worth investing in products that include them. Vitamin E is one of the most commonly included antioxidants in sunscreens and aftersun lotions. A formula that promises to be anti-ageing is a bonus because it should also contain anti-wrinkle ingredients. Some of these formulas not only protect the skin against burning, but also enhance its natural defence system. Vitamin E supplements can help boost the skin's defence system against ultraviolet rays and, if taken daily, can give your skin a protection equivalent to SPF4.

Waterproof sunscreens If you are planning to go on a very active, watersport-orientated holiday, choose a waterproof or a water-resistant sunscreen. Waterproof sunscreen should remain on the skin for up to 80 minutes before it needs to be reapplied and a water-resistant version should last for about 40 minutes. Research has shown that water dissolves the acid mantle (a thin protective layer) on the skin, leaving the skin more vulnerable to attack from the sun's rays. Because you will not feel yourself burning, be especially vigilant when you are in the water and make sure you reapply your suncream regularly.

Products for lips and eyes Lips and eyes are the most delicate areas of the face and require special protection in the sun. Combined lip and eye sticks are convenient to use and offer a high level of protection against UVA and UVB rays. Because the skin around the eyes is thinner than anywhere else on the face, this area is particularly vulnerable to burning and wrinkling. Make sure the entire eye area is covered lightly with a screen of at least SPF15 and always wear sunglasses.

Aftersun moisturizers All aftersun lotions moisturize and soothe the body, but some brands also include antioxidants, like vitamin E, and other ingredients that help keep the skin cells healthy and make them less prone to ageing. Many aftersun moisturizers also contain small amounts of fake tanning ingredients that give the skin a subtle boost of colour. Try to find one aftersun lotion that has been specifically formulated for use on the delicate skin of the face and then another, perhaps cheaper one, for use on the rest of the body.

sunscreens for sensitive skin

- Use physical blocks (titanium dioxide) instead of chemical sunscreens.
- Use a paba-free sunscreen. Paba is short for para-aminobenzoic acid and it can cause irritation to the skin and stain clothing.
- Don't use any anti-ageing products on holiday, especially fruit acids or retinol creams (see pages 214 and 218). Your skin's defences will be down because of the increased attack from the sun and you may overload it.
- If your skin is dry, choose a cream; if it is oily, opt for a light-textured lotion or gel. With the combination of heat and increased perspiration, a screen that is too heavy may cause irritation.

---

how to avoid a future face lift

DO protect your skin against wrinkle-forming UVA as well as burning UVB (look for a high SPF and the maximum four-star rating on the packaging).

DO wear a hat.

DON'T lie out in the sun at midday.

---

countdown to beauty

Several days before your holiday attend to all the important details that can make or break your naturally ravishing appearance. If you have forgone an exercise or anti-cellulite programme, now is the time to fake the rest.

Have your eyelashes and eyebrows dyed, and, if you want to be really organized and horrify friends with your vanity, have your lashes permed. Shaping the brows by thinning the outer lower part will also give your face a neater, fresher appearance – useful the morning after a long, alcoholic evening.

If you highlight your hair, talk to your colourist about having your hair done just before the holiday. If your hair has been bleached in any way, it will already be quite dehydrated and vulnerable to further attack from ultraviolet light, chlorine and sea water. Chlorine can turn bleached hair green, among a medley of other possible shades, although many of the newer hair dyes no longer just bleach the hair but replace it with other colour molecules that are far less likely to shift in shade significantly. However, whether your hair is dyed or not, you should expect it to go a few shades lighter when you expose it to strong sunlight.

This is also the perfect time to treat yourself to a good haircut, which will make it easier to style after a day on the beach. Also, have a deep conditioning treatment, which nourishes and protects the hair.

exfoliation

Using a body scrub, or having an exfoliation treatment in a beauty salon, is the quickest way to acquire glowing, healthy-looking skin. Body scrubs are now available in a variety of forms, from sea-salt rubs drenched in essential oils to high-tech grains blended with iridescent powder that leave the skin slightly shimmery. Choose whatever type, smell or packaging attracts you. The huge advantage of scrubs over loofahs or other traditional exfoliants is that the formulas include skin-softening and moisturizing ingredients. I have never understood the attraction of loofahs – they clog with dead skin cells in no time, attract hairs and are fantastically unhygienic after a few weeks. All scrubs should be used in a similar way: using firm, circular movements work from the extremities towards the heart.

depilation

Apart from electrolysis or laser hair removal, both of which are time-consuming and expensive, waxing is the best option for a smooth hair-free body (see also page 142). Although the first few times you have a bikini line waxed you will seriously question your sanity, waxing is well worth the pain. Hair regrowth is slow, at about four to six weeks, and you do not get rough stubble. Get legs, armpits, bikini line and moustache, if necessary, waxed. Do not be too alarmed if the skin bleeds a little after a bikini wax; it will heal in a matter of hours. If the skin feels tender, apply a little antiseptic cream for the next couple of days. Avoid hot baths the evening after having legs or a bikini line waxed or else the plundered follicles will turn bright red and take longer to calm down. Keep the waxed skin out of direct sunlight for 24 hours because too much heat will bring out redness. If skin becomes itchy or irritated, apply a little hydrocortisone cream (you can buy a gentle version from chemists), but do not use it if the skin is broken. Taking an antihistamine will also calm irritated skin.

fake a tan

Do not be tempted to use a pre-tan accelerator or tanning pills. These ultimately increase the chances of long-term damage to the skin. Your skin's defence against UVA is lowered and these methods can cause allergies and increase signs of ageing. Applying a little fake tan – or having it luxuriously applied for you in a beauty salon – is a great way of avoiding the luminous look when you first sally forth in your bikini. Not only will you feel more confident, but you will also be less vulnerable to overdoing sun exposure in an attempt to gain a bit of colour.

The whole concept of fake tans has changed dramatically in recent years. Terrible memories of turning from pale and pasty to bright ginger in a few hours still linger with most of us. Fake tans have been traditionally difficult to apply, extremely smelly and potentially humiliating. Effects were dramatic to say the least. I remember going to a party with legs that looked as if they had spent a month in the Caribbean while the rest of my body looked more like it had been on a driving holiday in France (fear and panic had set in halfway through the application process). Unlike wash- or wear-off tans or skin tints, which merely coat the surface of your skin with colour, the active ingredient in all fake tans, DHA (dihydroxyacetane), oxidizes the amino acid in the skin, turning it brown. Although this method has not really changed over the years, the results are far more natural these days, thanks to the other ingredients that are now included in the formulas.

In the age of skin-cancer awareness, fake tans are the intelligent and safe choice, and a vast choice of self-tanning formulas are now available, from wash-off colour to sunscreen with tanning ingredients added. There is something for everyone, whether taking the form of a mousse, gel, spray, lotion or liquid. There is also far more choice in terms of shade, and some are so subtle that no-one but you will notice – you will just look healthier. Textures also vary, such as oil-free versions for greasy skin, and many formulas are now tinted to help prevent any gaps in the colour during application. Formulas for the face even include antioxidant vitamins and skin-smoothing AHAs.

Modern self-tanners are also faster acting than the old versions, with some producing colour within an hour of application. Use a formula that is specifically for the face, as the shades will be more natural-looking and the product more gentle. Face self-tanners can be used on the body, but body self-tanners are not the best choice for the face.

applying fake tan

1. Remove dry and dead skin cells with an exfoliator so the fake tan applies evenly. On the face, use an exfoliator specified for the face or, for a home-made scrub, mix some caster sugar with a tiny amount of olive oil and massage it gently over the skin before rinsing off. On the body, use an exfoliator or body scrub (see page 28) and pay particular attention to the rough skin on the elbows and knees and around the heels.

2. Smooth or spray the fake tan onto moisturized skin following the manufacturer's instructions – some dry patches may soak up more colour than others.

3. For a natural look on the hands, keep your fingers together while you wipe the fake tan lightly across the backs of the hands.

4. Wash your palms well afterwards.

pack it in

Packing to go on holiday is almost always a stressful experience, usually done at 1 a.m. in a state of pre-holiday celebratory alcoholic stupor. Really organized people buy little Perspex containers and bottles into which they decant their beauty needs. Apart from the satisfaction of feeling smugly efficient and saving some, but not a great deal of, space, this is not really to be recommended. If you are going on a two-week holiday, you will just end up replenishing your supplies with a weird foreign product that smells of kitchen spray. Beware of flip-top lids – however fabulous the product may be inside, they often open and disgorge their contents. If you buy a flip-top product, put it in a plastic bag for packing.

beauty kit checklist

- ♥ Sunscreen for the face and another for the body.
- ♥ Two bottles of aftersun.
- ♥ A combined lip and eye block.
- ♥ Burn-soothing cream, such as calamine lotion or a simple dermatological cream.
- ♥ Frequent-wash shampoo and a rich protein conditioner.
- ♥ A combined make-up and mascara remover – the combined oil and water formulas are lighter than more traditional cleansers and are better in the heat.

- ♥ Antihistamine tablets for reducing inflammation and soothing rashes and insect bites.
- ♥ Cold/flu pills or powders.
- ♥ Bicarbonate of soda for a burn-relieving bath – add several tablespoons to the running water.

morning beauty routine

Whether you are on a luxury romantic tour of the Italian lakes or on a cheap and cheerful jolly with old friends, morning habits do not vary wildly. Eye bags will need to be deflated and soothed and the first steps towards the day's skin protection taken.

1. Sunscreen takes some time to sink into the skin, so apply a little in place of a moisturizer before breakfast. Do not confuse an SPF15 moisturizer with sunscreen. UV-screening moisturizer has really been formulated for everyday life, not powerful sunlight, and often offers no protection against UVA rays.

2. Reduce under-eye bags by applying a little astringent eye gel that has been kept in the fridge. Pat a pea-sized amount around the entire eye socket, or 'contour' as it is known in the trade. Alternatively, place a cold slice of raw potato over each eye. Thanks to the potassium content, potato is said to do wonders for dark circles.

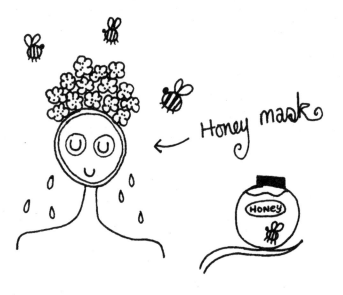

Honey mask →

HONEY

3. If your face feels really tight and dry, apply some runny honey or (preferably fresh) mayonnaise as a face mask. Leave it for 20 minutes before rinsing off.

4. If your hair feels very dry, brittle and damaged, mash up a ripe avocado and leave it on your hair for 30 minutes, then rinse thoroughly.

5. Do not spray on scent unless it is an alcohol-free version – the combination of alcohol and sunlight can cause staining on the skin.

6. Use your favourite perfume in deodorant form. Although it will not prevent you from sweating, it will contain antibacterial ingredients that kill off the germs that cause body odour. This is a good two-in-one product that will help save space.

---

how to look thin on the beach

Pick a spot where the sand is dry and uneven, and hollow out two leg-sized areas. Position your towel or sarong over the furrows, place a leg in each one and admire the fact that gravity prevents your thighs from spreading horizontally.

Never sit up straight. Always lie with your legs stretched out, with one knee bent for a relaxed, casual air, and your weight supported by your elbows. This lets you make eye contact with people, sip drinks and stare mysteriously out to sea without your stomach looking like the folds of a ruched blind.

---

health care

However tempting it is to see your bronzed face and body as a new healthy version of the dull putty original, sadly all dermatologists – especially those who specialize in sun-related skin problems – view a tan as damaged skin. The tan itself is the skin's defence system kicking in, preventing damage by turning brown. Preventing overexposure is the first step. However, damage to the skin can be reduced slightly by applying the right aftersun (see page 25). Some aftersun lotions can leave a very shiny residue, which will enhance redness if you are burnt, so choose one that offers a slightly matte finish.

Besides burning, there are other health issues you need to consider. As with any illness, if symptoms persist or worsen, contact the local physician or clinic.

Heat rash can be identified by the telltale little raised bumps that appear on the skin. If this happens, take some antihistamine and stay out of direct sunlight. Heat rash usually takes between one to four days to disappear.

Sunstroke is characterized by light-headedness, sleepiness and nausea. More serious symptoms include throbbing headaches and uncoordinated behaviour, and in this case contact a doctor immediately. Stay out of the sun, drink plenty of water and avoid alcohol. Cold compresses or towels placed over the body will also help.

An upset stomach is particularly distressing on holiday. A widely practised theory is that you should allow an upset stomach to heal itself, rather than taking pills. If your symptoms do not improve after three days, consult a doctor. One of the most common triggers – which has nothing to do with the state of hygiene in the local taverna – is quenching your thirst with freezing cold (particularly carbonated) drinks. If your body is hot, loading your stomach with cold liquid, then hurling yourself into cooler sea water or a swimming pool, is bound to make your stomach confused. Drink cool or even tepid water instead. Also, avoid drinking coffee and citrus-fruit juice or eating strong-tasting food. Eating rice, eggs, apricots and natural yoghurt always seems to help.

Dysentery is a different kettle of fish and a serious illness. Symptoms may include a high fever, headache, vomiting and stomach aches. Whereas ordinary diarrhoea lasts only a week or even less, dysentery can last considerably longer.

To ease a bloated stomach, avoid eating vegetables and fruit and substitute comfort food like mashed potato, cold soup and live yoghurt. Avoid any diet food, especially diet yoghurt, as it tends to swell in the stomach to give the impression of fullness. Other potential bloaters include carbonated drinks, pasta, bread and beans. Do not chew gum or drink from a bottle or through straws, all of which will make you swallow air.

If you have been dive-bombed by a bloodthirsty mosquito, apply calamine lotion or an antiseptic cream and take an antihistamine tablet. An added advantage is that the tablets will also help soothe any sunburn. If you are one of those unlucky people to whom mosquitoes are irresistibly drawn, use a sunscreen and aftersun lotion that includes a mosquito repellent in the formulas.

burn solutions

💜 If your face is burnt, a cold natural yoghurt face mask is soothing (see page 117). Alternatively, use an ordinary aftersun like a face mask, leaving it to soak in for about 10 minutes, then wiping off the rest with a tissue.

💜 Add several tablespoons of bicarbonate of soda to the bath for a burn-relieving soak.

💜 Stay out of the sun, drink plenty of fluids (preferably still, room-temperature mineral water) and rest quietly.

daytime make-up

Wearing ordinary make-up when you are on the beach is not recommended, unless you want to look like the Bride of Dracula after a swim. However, cosmetics companies have recently launched excellent stay-put mascara formulas and water-resistant (not waterproof) eyeshadows. Some have even come up with waterproof and sand-proof hair gel, which seem very imaginative from a marketing point of view. Although wearing waterproof mascara on your lashes and brows (choose the palest shade you can find for brows) is worth doing, the remaining contents of your make-up bag are best left for the evening.

Foundation does not offer enough protection for strong ultraviolet light. Even if the product claims an SPF15 protection, you are unlikely to put it on thickly enough to cover the skin completely. Likewise, blusher that claims to offer sun protection will do next to nothing, unless you wear it all over your face. However, if you are not intent on sunbathing and do want to wear some colour on your face, use a tinted moisturizer that contains sunscreen. Unless your skin is chalk-dry, choose an oil-free formula. Many clever new tinted moisturizers contain microsponges, which help absorb excess oil. An oil-free water-based sheer foundation is another alternative. Once it is applied to the skin, the water in the formula evaporates, giving an instant cooling sensation and leaving the skin shine-free.

If you must wear lip colour on the beach, choose a non-transfer formula in a natural shade. The drawback with many non-transfer formulas is that they tend to be drying, but slicking some ultraviolet-screening lip balm over the colour will remedy this. A less long-lasting choice is a natural coloured lip gloss that also offers sun protection.

evening make-up

The end of the day approaches and you finally acknowledge that if you lay on your beach towel for much longer it could be considered a skin graft. Relaxed and greasy, you head off for the pre-evening preparations. After a shower and a generous application of aftersun, attend to cosmetic needs. Make-up with a tan is always tricky and even modest amounts can look excessive in the heat. Use an oil-free foundation or tinted moisturizer (see daytime make-up, page 39) or dab a little concealer where needed. If you want to define your eyes but keep the look natural, use waterproof mascara and add a tiny bit of eyebrow pencil to the outer arches of the brows – do not fill in the entire brow. Put a tiny dot of a little pale eyeshadow on the middle of the eyelids and blend it across with your finger. Choose a sheer lip colour – avoid strong colours and heavy textures, which might clash with your tan or make you look tired.

holiday hair

Whether your fabulous new perm has turned into a Brillo pad or your strawberry-blonde streaks have combined with chlorine to match the salad, holiday hair can be a confidence basher. Humidity can make cascades of beautiful curls become frizz and limp hair become even thinner and limper. As far as hair is concerned, you will just have to look natural. However many sprays, gels and lotions you buy, you will probably find there is little you can do during the day about the style, but you can protect the hair from unnecessary damage.

Sun, sea and chlorine all weaken the hair and plunder its protein reserves so you will need to treat hair to far more nourishment than usual. Avoid using a hair dryer and invest in a rich hair mask, some of which are now formulated to help repair sun-damaged hair. You do not need to spend money on expensive sunscreens specifically made for use on the hair, just comb your normal sunscreen through your tresses. Many of the latest formulas now come as sprays, which means they can just as easily be applied to the hair as to the body. You could also mix your ordinary sunscreen with conditioner and leave it in your hair all day. Alternatively, add a little oil-free sunscreen to a pump-action (rather than aerosol) hair spray, shake well to mix it, then spritz it over your hair when you need it.

sightseeing

There is a point in most holidays when lolling around, staring at your toenails silhouetted against the horizon becomes boring. The moment to go and 'see' something arrives. If you are in a hot climate, this is prime burning time and yet a great opportunity to be just a little bit more alluring than you otherwise might, lying by the pool tucking into your fifth ice cream of the day.

The best look for cultural moments is '*English Patient* meets *Indiana Jones*' – a blend of cool, classic elegance (linen, beige and white are the key clothing colours) with flat, comfortable shoes. Unless you are very sure-footed, wearing sandals to go exploring means toe-stubbing becomes inevitable, which is not great for cultivating an alluring walk or preserving beautifully pedicured feet. Sunblock and a hat are a necessity for climbing ruins in the

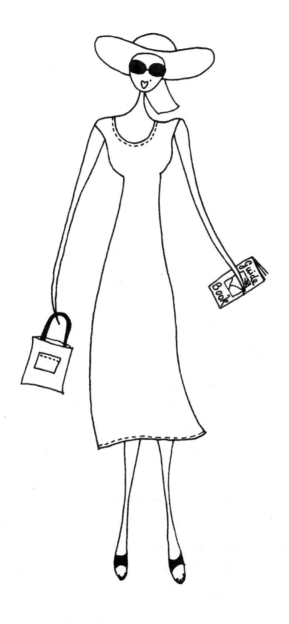

the summer holiday

sun. If the combination of heat, perspiration and increased heartbeat (caused by beautiful sights, walking uphill or a moment alone with the holiday Romeo) leave you looking like a greasy radish, wear a physical (titanium dioxide) sunblock for the face (see pages 23–4). Although these blocks once left a white, chalky finish on the skin, the particles are so finely milled in the latest formulas that they are undetectable and also leave the skin shine-free. If they give any colour, it is usually a very slight whitening effect, which is handy if you have a tendency to flush easily in the heat. If you want to wear some sort of foundation or tinted moisturizer, choose an oil-free, oil-absorbing formula to fight the grease-ball glow of heat and perspiration.

Cultural interludes are also fantastic opportunities to sneak off for beauty treatments, especially if you have a kindred spirit on holiday with you. That way, you can both slink around in the evening looking beautifully groomed and pretend that you went to see a thrilling old basilica, when you were actually having a relaxing massage and manicure in the nearest beauty parlour.

jungle beauty

Tropical climates have a special set of hazards. Trekking through an Asian jungle in my twenties was an unmitigated beauty disaster. I smelt, my skin turned from dry peaches and cream to red and greasy and I sprouted spots. The solution was simple: in humid climates you barely need moisturizer, but if you do, use an oil-free formula. Wear a sunscreen gel rather than cream to help reduce the grease factor. Toner is essential and will prevent your pores from being plugged with grime as well as keep you feeling clean against all the odds. For a less expensive alternative to a branded toner, buy witch hazel from a chemist, asking them to mix it with rose-water if your skin is sensitive.

Make-up is best avoided. If eyelashes are dyed and eyebrows shaped, you will look dazzlingly groomed anyway. Also, there is something mildly tragic about using make-up remover in an equatorial rainforest.

Sprinkling some talcum powder inside your shoes will instantly make your feet feel more comfortable and counteract unattractive smells at the end of a day. Also, make sure you have some antihistamine and hydrocortisone cream with you for emergencies. If you are bitten by monster mosquitoes, sucked by leeches or find the whole experience so petrifying you break out in hives, you will need something to calm your skin and counter an over-enthusiastic immune system.

sporty glamour

Summer sports activities are fabulous body toners and should be encouraged at most opportunities. I do, however, remember my heart sinking a little when a travelling companion looked up water sports in a Venice guide book. Perhaps he thought jet-skiing down the Grand Canal had a certain aftershave-advertisement glamour. The following pointers should ensure a higher beauty level than might otherwise occur.

Always wear plenty of waterproof or at least water-resistant sunblock. If you are water-skiing, wind-surfing or boogie-boarding, tie your hair off your face – not only will

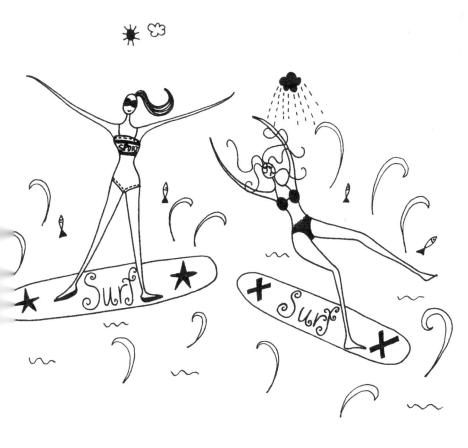

you be able to see better, you will also look more like a mermaid than the Loch Ness monster if you fall over. If the weather is hot enough to water-ski without a wetsuit, wear cycling shorts or two swimming costumes – this will help avoid giving yourself an enema if you fall over violently.

No-one's face ever looks good when diving with a regulator in their mouth or a mask clamped over the nose and lips, so just forget what you look like and concentrate on sub-aqua safety. Also remember that noses tend to run vigorously after swimming and general water sports activities, so check your nose is globule free before being within scrutiny of others.

look better that you really do

- ❤ DO use sunscreen that also contains fake tan. In just a day you will develop a pretty, golden glow and be beautifully protected against burning.
- ❤ DO drink litres of mineral water (preferably still rather than carbonated) and delight in the fact that you are giving your body a fabulous detoxing treatment.
- ❤ DON'T wear swimming costumes with frilly ruffles around the leg holes. They do not cover up fat legs and may make hips look bigger.
- ❤ DO wear a sarong around your hips at every opportunity.
- ❤ DO use an aftersun with a tan prolonger/enhancer included to maximize golden skin without damage.

♥ DO comb a sunscreen through your hair in the morning and reapply at lunchtime.

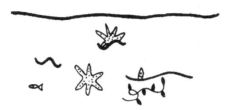

♥ DO use sand to scrub dead skin away. Sit at the water's edge, and use handfuls of wet sand as a body scrub. Use small circular movements from your feet up to the tops of your legs.

chapter two

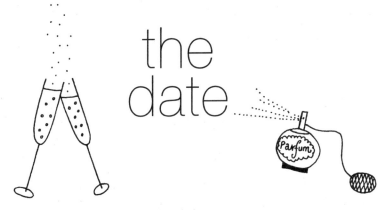

the date

Few things are as high risk to natural beauty as a date. Nervous rashes, spots and even cold sores seem to have an uncanny knack of appearing like parents at teenage parties. They arrive at the very moment you plan to metamorphose into a creature drenched in feline charm and beauty – and expose you as the human you really are. An irresistible temptation is to ladle on more make-up to compensate for a lack of confidence or to refuse to make any effort at all because seeming 'too keen' is a sign of weakness and will make you feel vulnerable if the date goes badly. 'I'm not going to bloody wash my hair,' snorted a friend of mine. 'I don't want him to think I've tried too hard.' These anxieties are compounded by the fear of blushing (if the date appears too keen), colour draining from normally peachy cheeks (when he reveals his penchant for sado-masochism) and failing to keep calm and relaxed.

However tragic it may seem for women at the end of the twentieth century to get courage from something as trivial as cosmetics, they do work. I put this down to the idea that we are really rather simple cavewomen, daubing ourselves with plant extract in the hope that Tarzan will pitch up. The complication is that there are about a million things you can do and products you can try, and looking fabulous is no longer a simple matter of rolling around in papaya juice and chalk. Exfoliating, depilating, scrubbing and scenting yourself into oblivion may be rather clichéd ways of preparing for a date, but boosting your confidence will do more than give a superficial sense of beauty. In trying some health-orientated techniques, like those in this chapter, you will become an irresistible and serene siren.

keep cool

Reducing existing stress levels paves the way for a calmer, more alluring air and, in the long term, better skin and a healthier body, even if it is for your own benefit and no-one else's. To control crazed emotions, you need to understand what is going on in your body during moments of stress. Before a date, your hormones, if not your heartbeat, will be raging. Because we are basically the same creatures that once depended on adrenaline rushes to get us out of danger, we still respond to stress in the same way. If you are worried or even scared, adrenaline levels increase, blood pressure rises and breathing quickens. This overreaction mechanism in the body is known as the sympathetic system; the calming side is the parasympathetic system. To reduce natural stress levels, cut down on stimulants that throw the body's stress-regulating system out of whack. Poor diet, lack of exercise and irregular sleep patterns stress the body, eventually making it less robust and able to deal with stress. Consider the stereotypical workaholic who stays up all night, drinks and smokes like it is going out of fashion and then wonders why he or she feels burnt out at an early age. Helping your body remain as naturally calm as possible is the most beneficial course of action in the long term. Although the habits that contribute to stress are not going to disappear overnight, there are a few steps you can take in the short term to help you relax.

stress-coping techniques

- Cut out caffeine, nicotine and alcohol. This will reduce anxiety levels, improve your complexion and enhance your energy levels.
- Get adequate sleep.
- Go for a brisk walk for 20 minutes or more, trying to break into a slight sweat.
- Go to the gym for an hour rather than lying in front of the television fantasizing about your date and all the possible outcomes.
- For a quick pick-me-up just prior to the date, shake your hands vigorously from the wrists: this has an instantly calming effect.
- Massage the inner arch of the sole of the foot to help calm any pre-date nerves.
- Don't worry too much if you can't sleep the night before the date. When you are tired, your reactions are not as defensive nor your wit as sharp and, as we all know, most men like to feel in control.
- Try to think of yourself as a hopelessly attractive femme fatale, deciding whether you like the date, not the other way around.
- Comfort yourself with the knowledge that most men don't actually notice the specifics of your appearance. They are far more interested in how attractive they are appearing and the likelihood of winning you over.

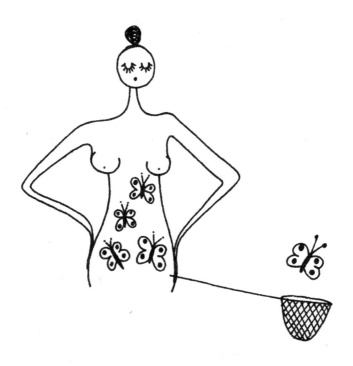

the plough

Yoga exercises will help relax the body and mind. The plough position is great for calming and stretching.

1. Lie on your back on the floor with your legs straight out.

2. Raise your legs into a shoulder stand, supporting the base of your spine with your hands.

3. Gently bend your legs over your head, keeping them straight while continuing to support your back.

4. Hold the position for as long as you feel comfortable, but for no more than five minutes. Keep your neck flat against the floor throughout.

5. Still supporting your back, slowly uncurl, bringing your legs to the floor. You may find it more comfortable and easy to uncurl one leg at a time.

holistic approaches

If you are feeling very jumpy, have a massage, preferably one that includes aromatherapy. Not only will you feel luxuriously indulged and pampered, but you will also have been given a 'healing hands' treatment and physical reassurance is a powerful confidence builder. In addition to relieving knotted muscles, most massage leaves you feeling more mentally relaxed. One beauty therapist I interviewed told me that some of her clients cry when they are massaged because it releases so much tension. Because certain essential oils can help increase relaxation or energy levels, combining aromatherapy with massage will help bring frazzled nerves to heel.

For home relaxation invest in aromatherapy products, such as scented candles, massage oils, bath oils or smelling salts – even a cassette of dolphins whistling might help. Lip glosses flavoured with essential oils to lift or relax the spirits of the wearer are also worth a try.

Aromatherapists swear by lavender oil as one of the best relaxers. If you are overexcited and cannot sleep the night before a date, put a few drops of lavender oil on a tissue near your pillow. Drink camomile tea before bed and try some slow yogic breathing (see page 13) to help you relax. This deep breathing technique will come in handy as a quick calmer when you are on the date, but practise doing it as noiselessly as possible. A deep throaty grunt could minimize your chances.

aromatherapy bath oils

Adding three to five drops of an essential oil to a warm bath will help prepare you for the big event mentally and physically. Have a bath in low light and with candles or soft music to intensify the experience.

- ❤ For a fatigued brain: patchouli, basil, cypress or peppermint oils.
- ❤ For a bad case of nerves: sage, lavender, basil, jasmine or juniper oils.
- ❤ For resentment (if he is late or has blown you out on a previous date): rose oil.
- ❤ For lack of confidence and general feelings of weakness: camomile, melissa or jasmine oils.
- ❤ For grumpiness: lavender, camomile, marjoram or frankincense oils.

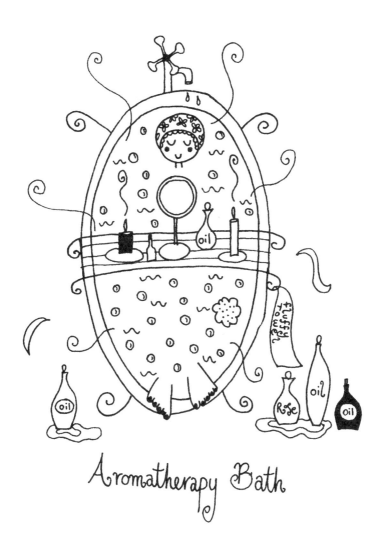

Aromatherapy Bath

pre-date beauty tips

- DO invest in a swanky new piece of make-up. A good concealer is always indispensable and can be hidden discreetly in a handbag.
- DON'T experiment with unfamiliar or time-consuming beauty treats, such as face packs or exfoliators.
- DON'T try a new hairdresser or a radically new haircut.
- DON'T have a makeover at a cosmetics counter. Unless you hit a rare make-up talent, at best you will walk away feeling overly made-up and at worst you will look like you are auditioning for a transvestite part in the *Rocky Horror Picture Show*.
- DO have a manicure at a salon or at home. This pampering treat will help take your mind off your nerves.

cosmetic charm

A universally acknowledged truth is that when a woman reaches a certain age, she needs make-up. I am not suggesting that you should charge off to a beauty counter at the nearest department store and squander most of your mortgage deposit on an array of cosmetics for every part of your face. There are, however, are a few fantastic beauty supports that really are worth having, such as a sheer, natural-looking foundation, a good concealer and a nude lipstick.

When I was working on *Cosmopolitan*, we tried to write a feature on what men thought of make-up – whether they found watching girls putting it on sexy, whether they liked red lips, heavily made-up eyes, or something else. The result was a non-piece. Men seemed to find plenty to hate but very little that interested them. Some areas of loathing were heavily glossed, strongly coloured lips, long dark nails and heavy eyeshadow. Overenthusiastically sprayed hair was another turn-off. The one unanimous opinion was that make-up was fine provided it was undetectable. The best approach is to look gloriously peachy-cheeked and radiant by wearing plenty of make-up but so cleverly applied that it is disguised. In other words, be the queen of fake but natural beauty.

Old ideas of make-up being a heavy mask worn by middle-aged women should have died out years ago. Although they do still persist, make-up gets better and more undetectable every year due to the new technology that is constantly being developed and improved and the amazingly competitive cosmetics market. Colours are far more subtle than they used to be because the pigments are now milled more finely, and the fluids that these pigments are suspended in are lighter. Also, cosmetics companies now cater for different skin types and tones, offering a huge choice in finishes, staying power and skin benefits in everything from foundation to lipstick. As far as date make-up choice is concerned, this is fantastic news.

getting the base-ics right

Foundation today is one of life's miracles. Years ago, the formulas were largely cement-like in consistency and the finish about as natural as Hollywood. The formulas tended to be wax-based, which felt heavy, or a colour-saturated cream, which gave an opaque, unnatural appearance. But over the last few years foundation has changed completely, and although keeping abreast of all the latest developments is a boring enough interest for even the most beauty-conscious, knowing what sort of formula to choose and how to apply it is fundamental to looking fabulously flawless and natural.

Now that there are more choices on the market than ever before, the biggest problem is selection. If you ask for help at a cosmetics counter, you will not simply be offered a choice of colour. A whole raft of new foundation selling words and phrases distinguish one type from another. The most important term to consider when choosing a foundation is 'texture'. You will probably be offered dewy, radiant, light-reflecting, matte or satin, to mention just a few. Of course choosing the right one is entirely a matter of personal preference, but all the textures basically reduce down to the following finishes: shiny or matte with heavy or light coverage. In my experience the best foundation for a beautiful glowing skin is a light, slightly moisturizing formula.

Light-reflecting pigments are another tremendous bonus for faking healthy skin. The pigments help bounce light away from the skin, like microscopic mirrors, giving the impression of a lovely, pearly glow. Although light-reflecting pigments have been around for years, a more recent development is found in foundations that offer 'photochromatic technology'. These formulas look entirely natural in all sorts of different light from daylight, which can render foundation very grey or fake-looking, to golden evening light. If the foundation formula contains volatile silicone (see page 246), this will also be a bonus. As a single ingredient, silicone has revolutionized cosmetics by giving them a silky feel and making them easier to apply. Volatile silicones allow the colour (or pigment) to glide on beautifully and then, because they are volatile, they evaporate, leaving the pigment welded to the skin. Water-based foundations operate in the same way, and because water cools as it evaporates, a lovely refreshing sensation can be felt as the foundation 'sets'.

cover up

There are almost as many varieties of concealers as there are foundations. Choose from light-reflecting, traditional matte finishes, or special versions for hiding scars and various skin complaints. Some formulas also include skin-care treatments for reducing dark circles or puffy eyes. If you do not have concealer, use the dehydrated foundation that accumulates around the top of the tube or bottle – it is almost the same. Apply concealer after foundation, otherwise the concealer will just be rubbed off.

Dark circles For dark circles, but not bags, under the eyes, choose a concealer that contains 'light-reflecting pigments'. The tiny particles in the pigment refract light off the skin. A traditional concealer is just a thicker version of foundation and will form into crepey lines under the eyes. Some eye creams for counteracting dark circles, especially those for daytime use, have light reflectors included in the formula. The light reflectors make black circles reduce in strength almost instantly, tricking you into believing that the cream is getting rid of the dark circles when it is really only disguising them.

To cover up circles, face the mirror, tilt your chin down slightly and look up: the worst part of the dark rings will be visible. Using a brush or your ring finger, apply a little concealer in this area only and blend it in gently. If you apply concealer where the rings look their worst when you look straight into the mirror, or you try to cover the entire under-eye area, you will create 'panda eyes'.

Red veins or burst capillaries Do not use green or blue concealer or foundation, however much the packaging may claim they are the perfect solution. Unless you are a professional make-up artist, they are difficult to apply and rarely look natural. Green, in particular, can give a terrible grey tinge. Instead, dab on a little moisturizing concealer, gently rocking it into the skin with your finger.

Birthmarks Choose a heavy-duty concealer specially formulated to cover scars and birthmarks (see page 198). Some versions are even waterproof.

Spots Choose a concealer specifically formulated for covering up and drying out spots. Moisturizing concealers will not help reduce spots and the light-reflecting formulas will only emphasize them. If you cannot find a spot concealer, dab a little witch hazel or toner on the spot and then paint the concealer on with a brush. Use powder applied with a cotton bud to set the concealer – the powder will make the spot less likely to catch the light.

transfer-proof make-up

If you want to avoid the 'lipstick on the collar' effect, these formulas are good choices and available as foundations and blushers as well as lipsticks. Transfer-proof foundation tends to give chalky results and dehydrate the skin slightly, so even if you have flawless skin, the results may make you look tired. Lines under the eyes may also seem exaggerated by the slightly powdery finish. The same problems are encountered with transfer-proof lipstick. Once the initial sheen wears away, a matte, sometimes quite drying and unnatural-looking 'stain of colour' is left.

If skin tends to be greasy, a long-lasting formula might be perfect for you and many are oil-free. If you like matte rather than glossy lips, a long-lasting formula will also suit you. For normal to dry skins, these formulas are probably best used on specific occasions only and extra moisturizer or lip balm slicked on to counter any drying effects.

faking a healthy glow

Impressing your date with a luminous radiant glow is the easiest thing in the world to fake. If you are looking tired and all the light-reflecting pigments in the world are failing you, brush a little matte (not sparkly) pink eyeshadow or blusher underneath your eyes. This may sound like a make-up tip for an extra in a horror movie, but it is one of the oldest tricks in the book.

For a healthy-looking, glowing complexion, brush a little powder, or even a very light bronzer that has a slightly pearlized effect, very thinly all over the face. If you need more colour, brush the most boringly natural, matte powder blusher across the forehead, down over the nose and on the cheeks. Alternatively, blend a little cream blusher on the apples of the cheeks under foundation. This gives a bright and breezy look and is used by make-up artists all the time. New cream blushers are so subtle that they leave just a little stain of colour and the skin looks healthy, not overpowdered.

radiant skin round-up

- ❤ Apply double the usual amount of moisturizer under the foundation and spend at least a minute massaging it in all over the face, including under the chin, which can look dry.
- ❤ Wear a sheer, moisturizing, light-reflecting foundation.
- ❤ Avoid using matte, oil-free foundation, unless your skin is very greasy.
- ❤ Only apply foundation where it is needed, not all over the face, and blend it thoroughly.
- ❤ For extra coverage, build up tiny layers of foundation in specific areas. Applying one thick layer will not look as natural or be as effective.
- ❤ Don't wear powder. Because foundations 'set' themselves on the skin, they don't need holding in place with powder as well.
- ❤ Never wear powder directly under the eyes: it will crease and give you tiny lines, even if your skin is naturally pebble-smooth.
- ❤ Don't wear mascara or eyeliner on the lower eyelashes: it can make you look tired.
- ❤ On the date, make sure you sit with your back to the

strongest light source. You can then scrutinize the date's open pores without fear of the same being done to you.

💜 Avoid any date venue with bright, overhead lighting. The reason cheap fast-food joints are lit so brightly is to keep customers rotating: you can't relax in a brightly lit room, nor do you look your best.

---

how to avoid lipstick on wine glasses

Don't wear lipstick or lip gloss. Colour in the lips with a lip pencil in a natural shade instead.

💜

Lick your lips before taking a sip.

---

bright-looking eyes

1. Dab tiny dots of a neutral highlighter or pale concealer on the outer and inner corners of both eyes, using only a pinprick amount on the inner corners. Blend it in well with the tip of your little finger. This will lift the eyes and make them look brighter.

2. Cover the entire eyelid, up to the brow bone, with a neutral colour that is as close to your natural skin colour as you can find. This will open up the eyes and make any mottled areas or veins disappear.

3. Brush a layer of mascara over the top of the upper lashes, then twice from below. This gives definition, yet looks more natural than a thick third layer.

4. Add a very fine line of dark brown or grey eyeliner close to the upper lashes. Keep the liner subtle, or the fresh-faced, bright-eyed façade will be ruined.

hair flair

I have heard it said that, in Los Angeles, men who have extra-marital affairs choose women who have longer hair than their wives. Perhaps this is because women tend to cut their hair short when they have children or that they lead busy lives and do not have time to spend hours turning into a Barbie Doll. The bottom line is that loose locks, rather than a pinned-up librarian style, win the day. Loose hair is universally considered more sexy, which is great news if you have naturally thick hair. However, if you suffer from limp, fine hair, use a body-building spray close to the roots, spraying in more than you think you need, then comb it through and dry the hair upside down.

Now is definitely not the time to experiment with a new haircut or high-tech perm, or 'form' as some beauty salons now call it. Perms still have to grow out and that could leave you looking like a backing singer for a faded 1970s pop group for some time to come. There are few things as demoralizing as a hairstyle you hate. Make sure your hair is as glossy, healthy and 'touchable' as it can be.

date nails

There is nothing more unnecessary or revolting than dirty, chipped, witch-like nails. Keep nails shaped, but fairly short; you do not want to snag one and leave it hanging on your date's jumper. A friend of mine once suffered the humiliation of losing one of her nail tips in a pizza she had made for a sexy supper date: he found it in his mouth.

Do not wear long or false nails covered in vampy colours, unless you think your future boyfriend secretly hopes you are a porn star. To appear the wholesome, sweet creature you would like to be treated as, choose clear polish or a very pale pink or beige colour.

scent sense

Choosing a scent is one of life's most extraordinary and complicated decisions. Research shows that women no longer have just one 'signature scent' that they wear every day of the week regardless of the season and the occasion. Nor, thanks to the mid-1990s trend for more

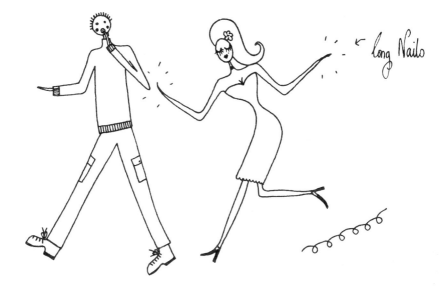

long Nails

subtle, light perfumes, should we be bound by the old rule that only tarts wear perfume before lunch.

Advertising has bombarded us with a hundred and one images that conjure up how we might feel and be if we wear a particular perfume. Although we all buy into labels to a certain extent, finding the right scent is one of the most subjective reflexes you can have. Perfumers and experts say that smell is our most ancient sense, and the smell information centre in the brain is closely located to the memory and 'pleasure' zones. This could explain why some smells repulse us for no discernible reason, while others fill us with pleasure.

When it comes to romance, scent can be immensely thrilling. If your date loves the way you smell and you genuinely love the scent you are wearing, there is a wonderful physical connection. However, do not read too much into this. If you think your date is quite the most fabulous creature imaginable, but he wears revolting aftershave, do not despair. Either he has an endearingly bad sense of style, no sense of smell or there are some – or even just one – ingredients, or 'notes', in the fragrance that trigger a bad memory for you. Perhaps, for example, cedarwood reminds you of a cologne-drenched physics teacher at school.

The scent you choose to wear can be open to misinterpretation. 'If I take a girl out and she smells really sophisticated and sexy, I'll know she's pretty keen,' leered one character I spoke to on the subject. So if you do not want to give the game away or inadvertently lead your date up the garden path, choose a more subtle, less statement-laden, scent for a first date. If, however, you are keen as mustard on him but have only secured the date by a covert plan and want to ensure his affection, consider the results of an American survey that monitored penile blood flow in relation to various aromas. The smell of pumpkin pie was revealed to be the most exciting and cookies were a close runner-up. Perhaps the smell of Christmas pudding would act as an aphrodisiac on British males. If you do want to pursue this line, you are in luck, because the latest sexy, warm and fruity perfumes are not a million miles away in notes from the aroma of a traditional warm winter pudding.

where to wear scent

Although all good Hollywood movies show femme fatales dabbing scent behind their ears, this is actually the wrong place to put perfume. A higher than average number of oil ducts are found around the ears and they can significantly alter or even suppress the true character of a particular scent. Other pulse points, such as wrists and behind knees, are better locations. Hair holds scent beautifully, so spray a little in your hair for a subtle fragrance.

daytime date

Daylight hours are always a challenge, especially in winter when light is cruel, blue and makes skin look pasty. Unless your natural colouring is blue-toned (very pale white skin, usually with black hair), you need to counteract the blue light with peachy-toned make-up. Applying a very sheer tawny-coloured blusher where the sun naturally hits the face will have an instant warming effect. Bronzer will look fake in winter, but can be applied like blusher during summer months when the light is warmer.

Most of us have yellow-toned skin, rather than pink, and a golden-toned foundation or concealer will 'disappear' once it has been blended well into the skin, making it undetectable in daylight. If you look tired, do not layer on make-up to compensate. Dab foundation on only in the places where you need it, such as over unevenly coloured skin, veins or blemishes, and blend it in smoothly. Use a moisturizing foundation to give the skin extra radiance.

last-minute date

You have just five minutes to metamorphose from a smelly, greasy warthog into a serene princess with poise and grace – this is the ultimate 'faking it' challenge. Employ some quick fixes (see opposite) on problem areas if necessary. Above all, be decisive and methodical and do not experiment with anything new.

💗 Suggest a dim and dark place to go for a drink.

💗 Dab on foundation and blusher or bronzer (see pages 62–3). Doing this in double-quick time will heat you up enough to give skin a natural, alluring glow.

💗 Forget the shower, but use deodorant and scent.

💗 Pulling hair off the face will make you look fresh-faced and clean, even if you don't feel it.

💗 If your nail polish is chipped, remove the colour and go nude. Trying to patch up the chips at the last minute will only look messy.

💗 Slick eyebrows into line with a tiny bit of moisturizer – it makes a remarkable difference, instantly refreshing the face and enhancing the eyes.

💗 Apply your favourite lipstick and a touch of gloss.

quick fixes: emergency action

For greasy hair: Scatter dry shampoo, talc or cornflour very finely near the roots. Massage it in to absorb the grease, then brush it out. Do not wear a black top.

For spots: Dab on any sort of astringent or alcohol, whether perfume, gin or proper antiseptic. Pat on a tiny bit of concealer and cover with a dab of powder.

For dry lips: Smother on lip gloss or salve, but not moisturizer. Lipstick will make the flakes look worse.

For dry skin: Dab the face with damp cotton wool, then apply petroleum jelly or an unscented lip salve directly to the skin. Applying foundation on a dry patch will only emphasize the dryness.

For a pale face: Splash with cold water 10 times, then hold your head upside down and count to 10. Apply a pinky blusher (if you can't find one, use lipstick) on the apples of the cheeks under foundation for a fake glow.

For smelly breath: Chew some parsley or suck on a blob of toothpaste while applying your make-up.

the morning after

Years ago, a men's magazine ran a feature on how to stock your bathroom for girls without them knowing. The article made fabulous reading and struck a chord, given that most men's bathrooms are either stiff-upper-lip shrines to the days of the Empire with nothing more than a razor, flared shaving brush, shaving soap, toothbrush and a stick of deodorant or they are a hair-covered, slime and gunge collection of glamorous ex-girlfriends' creams (all far more expensive than you can afford).

If you do find yourself in an alien bathroom the morning after a date, there will probably be a few products you can use effectively. All you really need is some sort of emollient cream for cleansing and moisturizing – even a bit of old aftersun will do. Or ask your date if he has some petroleum jelly. This may make you raise your eyebrow if he keeps it with a collection of magazines and leather accessories in a bedroom drawer, but otherwise, fall upon it like a long-lost friend. In its pure state, petroleum jelly is extremely unlikely to cause any sort of irritation so can be used safely close to the eyes and all over the face. Warm the petroleum jelly on the back of your hand first, then use it as a cleanser, eye make-up remover, moisturizer and lip salve.

If you are really stuck, you can even use petroleum jelly in place of make-up by putting a tiny bit on your lips, the top of your eyelids and on your cheekbones to catch the light. Finally, use it to slick your eyebrows into shape. Hair conditioner can also be used as a body moisturizer – you might even be lucky enough to find a conditioner that doubles up as a body cream anyway. It is a good idea to do a little 'patch test' first, though, because some conditioners leave a sticky film.

Check the kitchen for ingredients you can use as emergency beauty treatments. Olive oil and salt, or salt alone, can be used as a body scrub with a dry flannel. For an instant glow, mix together some honey and salt and rub it gently over your face, rinse it off and then splash your face several times with cool water.

If you cannot find any useful products at all, simply splash your face repeatedly with very cold water to improve your circulation, deflate eye bags and create a fresh-faced angelic-looking complexion.

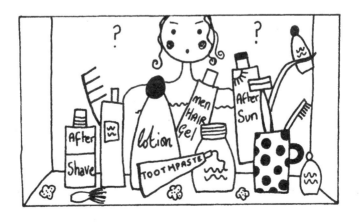

morning-after face massage

1. Press firmly on either side of your nose with your index fingers.

2. Move your fingers out along your eyebrows, pressing firmly, finishing at your temples. Repeat four times along each brow.

3. Apply a little pressure at the temples with your fingertips.

4. Press along your upper gum line.

strategies for stubble rash

If the skin on your face is grazed from a night of passionate kissing, practise the following tips:

- ❤ DON'T touch the sore skin.
- ❤ DO treat it with dermatological cream or petroleum jelly – an antiseptic cream could dry out the skin.
- ❤ DO keep moisturizing the rash by reapplying the cream regularly, even after a scab forms.
- ❤ DO cover the rash with a little powder – concealer and foundation are too heavy and might irritate the skin.
- ❤ DON'T let an unshaven chin near the wound.
- ❤ DON'T use an alcohol-based antiseptic unless you are

worried the graze might become septic. The antiseptic will sting badly and make the rash redder.

❤ DO dab on a little tea tree oil if the rash feels itchy.

the second date

Retain your mysterious air; you do not want to appear a reliable or predictable someone who does not offer much variety. At the same time, be extremely wary about changing your appearance radically. Your date is trying to get to know the real you and conflicting images may stump him. Always keep skin radiant and glowing (see page 63), but do something slightly different, perhaps make a subtle change in the way you style your hair, use a darker or lighter lipstick, or a smudge of slate-grey eyeshadow on the outer corners of your eyelids. Alternatively, you could use this opportunity to carry out a personality text, wearing fake tattoos or strange transfers on your nails and gauging his approval by nostril flare or upper-lip stiffening.

chapter three

the skiing holiday

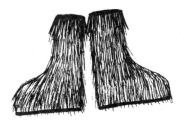

Skiing holidays are deceptively unglamorous. Of course, we have all seen pictures of nipped and tucked film stars swaggering around celebrity-packed resorts, and the mind does not have to leap far to imagine ourselves looking similarly fabulous. If the fantasy is being a 1960s-style snow siren, complete with white fur-trimmed accessories, Sophia Loren-style eye make-up and appropriately frosted pink lipstick, the reality is that most ordinary mortals skid nervously through icy resorts, the likes of which the Gstaad gang would not dream of being anywhere near. We end up looking more like boiled beetroots stuffed into anoraks than alluring double agents in a James Bond film.

Skiing is a physical and mental battlefield. Skin takes a hammering from the elements, your body is under stress from physical exertion and you will be emotionally charged from adrenaline rushes, having a ridiculously good time and, possibly, romantic encounters.

Faking your way through this minefield, from hearty, red-faced skier to mysteriously cool resort princess, is actually surprisingly easy. You just have to prepare yourself in advance and stick resolutely to the skiing holiday beauty tips on the following pages.

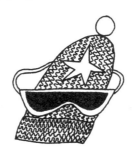

health and fitness

Two months before the holiday is the crucial time to begin getting in shape. The chances are you have stumped up a terrifying amount of money to go skiing and are beginning to think, but not necessarily do anything, about fitness. Talk to any sports physiotherapist or fitness instructor and they will tell you that making sure your limbs are strong and stable is more important than being aerobically fit. This is particularly true if you have ever suffered from any ligament or muscle injuries.

The muscles that need the most work are obviously those in the legs – the thighs and knee ligaments should be particularly sturdy. Because carrying skis can kill you off before you even reach the slopes, strengthening the arms is also important and will help you pull yourself up slopes after deviously skiing off-piste in the hope that a handsome hero will follow you – 'just to make sure you are safe'.

However much you hate going to a gym, try enrolling in a pre-ski class. Most gyms offer them and even if you hate looking at the contracting buttocks of your classmates, you can learn some good exercises and practise them at home. It is important to learn how to exercise safely and effectively to avoid causing muscle strain or injury. Skiing will make you stiffer than you have ever been before, but a couple of months of weekly classes will make your week of action much easier and consequently more enjoyable.

foot note

Book a chiropody checkup if you suffer from calluses, bunions or corns. Ski boots are notoriously uncomfortable, and if you have any problems with hard skin or painful toenails, now is the time to attend to them. Under no circumstances should you undergo a chiropody treatment less than a week before your holiday: nothing is worse than skiing with a raw toe.

From a beauty point of view, chiropody is also worth doing. Ugly, sore feet may remain hidden in thick woollen socks and ski boots during the day, but the chances are you will reveal them walking carelessly barefoot around the chalet in the evenings. You may also be spurred into having steam or sauna treatments, and while sweetly swollen feet after a day in ski boots are one thing, barnacled feet are quite another.

Make sure you see a qualified chiropodist – an unqualified one or an overenthusiastic pedicurist can actually do more harm than good (see listing on page 253). Chiropody usually involves the use of somewhat frightening skin-smoothing instruments. During a session, all the hard skin on the feet and toes is gently shaved away with little sharp scalpels. Although this sounds a potentially painful and terrifying experience, a good chiropodist should not cause even the slightest tinge of pain. Any tender skin is protected by an ordinary plaster for a couple of days.

pre-ski leg strengthener

If you cannot get to a gym, this is one of the best and simplest leg strengtheners.

1. Stand close to a wall, then lean back against it.

2. Bend your knees a little, no more than 45 degrees, and hold the position for as long as possible.

3. To make the exercise more difficult, hold your arms out straight ahead of you and hold it for up to 20 counts.

pre-ski tips

- ❤ DO book pre-ski classes at the local gym.
- ❤ DON'T engage in a frenzied bout of exercise at the last minute. You may end up straining muscles and being unable to ski.
- ❤ DO book chiropody checks for bunions and calluses.
- ❤ DO buy SPF25 sunscreen with the maximum four-star UVA filter.
- ❤ DO buy a combined lip and eye block.
- ❤ DO invest in a good pair of goggles or sunglasses.
- ❤ DON'T go on a sunbed 'to get your skin used to ultraviolet light': sunbeds do nothing for the skin's health and speed up the ageing process.

- ❤ DO get a good haircut and deep conditioning treatment.
- ❤ DO dye your lashes and eyebrows. This will pay dividends when you remove your sunglasses at lunch and will also help perk up your face for your early-morning airport start.

skin protection

Even if you are a hardened summer sun worshipper, do not make the mistake of thinking the same sun protection rules apply when you are on a skiing holiday. Ultraviolet light in mountains is unbelievably powerful, even on cloudy days. Not only are you at higher altitude, but the reflection from the snow increases the power and potentially damaging effects of the sun. Skin that is resilient in the summer months can suffer terrible burns and damage in the snow. I learnt this the hard way when I burnt my face so badly and it swelled to such proportions that I was called 'potato face' by my kind friends.

Skiing is a skin destroyer. Aside from the fact that you are treating yourself to some of the cleanest air on earth, skin takes a beating from the ice, snow, dehydration and extremes of temperature. Some of the mountain restaurants are so hot and steamy that it is surprising people can bear to wear any clothes in them at all.

When your face gets very cold, the fats or lipids that keep it looking and feeling comfortable and moisturized freeze, rather like wet clothes on a washing line on a cold winter's day. Tiny little fissures and cracks appear and water loss speeds up. If you have even a flicker of a peaches-and-cream complexion, you are particularly vulnerable – especially as this skin tends to be dry in the first place. Rosy cheeks become mini networks of burst capillaries, but this happens over years.

Of course you cannot control the outside temperature or the air and snow hitting your face, but you can prevent water from escaping unnecessarily from the skin by wearing a good moisturizer or petroleum jelly, as well as sunblock, over the rosy parts of your face. Some luxurious moisturizers promise to protect the skin from extremes of temperature. This claim seems ambitious to me, but some face creams have been beneficial to those testing them in Arctic conditions.

skin complaints and sensitivity

Eczema sufferers should be especially careful while skiing. Too high a dose of hydrocortisone cream combined with ultraviolet rays can have disastrous consequences – in my case it caused oversensitivity and an allergic reaction, which lasted for months afterwards. Because ultraviolet light usually helps calm eczema, stopping your steroid cream a few days before skiing and keeping off it until you return may be the best course of action.

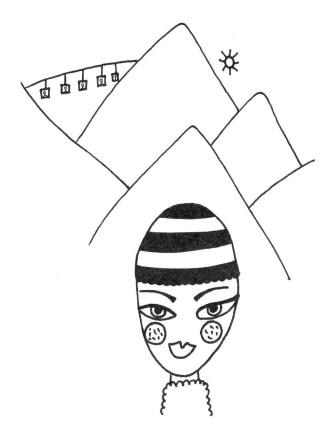

Also be wary of using certain acne drugs, retinol, AHAs or BHAs, or any other anti-ageing skincare products. Your skin will be taking a beating from the elements and there is no need to overload it. If you suffer from photosensitivity generally, it may be caused by antibiotics, antihistamines or even antidepressant pills. If you are at all worried, discuss your skin with your doctor before you go. Do not feel your concerns are trivial – your skin is the biggest organ in your body, so it deserves proper respect. You can minimize burning, rashes and other sun allergies by wearing a sunblock specially formulated for sensitive skins, though you may not find one specifically for skiing – make sure it is at least SPF25.

sunscreen

Invest in a sunscreen or block that is specifically for use at high altitude – most feature little pictures of mountains. Buy as small a tube as you can find (more than one if necessary) so you can carry it in your pocket. I would recommend a soft tube rather than a bottle because it will not be as painful if you fall on it. For very dark skins, an SPF15 is acceptable, but anyone else should start with at least SPF25. Higher factors will certainly do no harm.

Now that skin cancer and the ageing effects of the sun are so well recognized, wearing sunscreen is not just necessary to protect skin by preventing burns but also to preserve skin. Cosmetics companies have got the 'protective' ground reasonably covered and are moving into skincare in the sun as an extra benefit. If you choose a sunscreen that also includes antioxidants (see page 24) and other skincare ingredients, you will be treating, rather than simply protecting, your skin. Many 'vitamin' or antioxidant formulas are marketed as pollution protectors but they also help from within to protect the skin from excessive damage. If you have sensitive skin, choose a physical sunscreen, one that includes titanium dioxide in its ingredients, rather than a chemical formula (see also pages 23–4).

lip and eye care

Lips need special protection. If you are prone to cold sores, a skiing holiday may trigger them because you are in bright light (most likely at a time of year when you have been exposed to relatively little) and you will be tired and at times nervous if you are pushing yourself on the slopes. Wear protective lip salve, carry cold-sore cream at all times and avoid frightening slopes. Start taking an amino acid supplement, lysine, a month before you go. Lysine seems to be one of the best ways of suppressing cold sores.

Protecting your eyes is also extremely important. Unless you have skin like rhino hide, never ski in ordinary sunglasses. Wear proper ski sunglasses that offer UVA and UVB protection. Ideally they should cover the entire eye area, fitting over the eye sockets so no light can sneak in. Wearing sunblock over the eye area does not seem to work because perspiration makes it run into the eyes and sting. The best way to bump up protection around the eyes is with an SPF15 lip salve. Some ski lip salves are formulated for the eye area too.

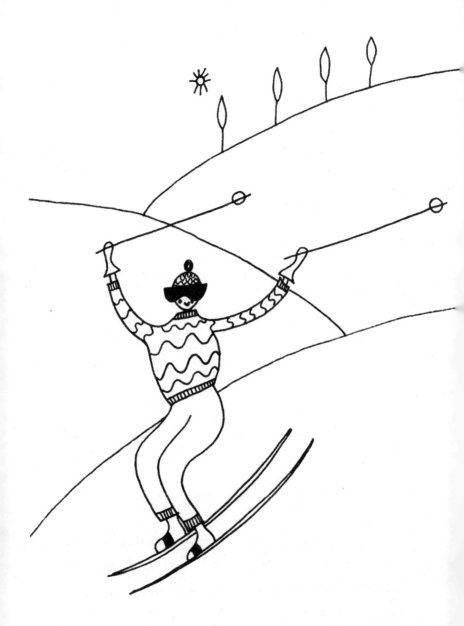

86 **the skiing holiday**

lift pass

♥

When you are looking your most ravishing, get your photograph taken for your lift pass. Although an exceptionally nauseating necessity, you will be glad to have a reminder of your other gorgeous self when you are smothered in sunblock in a steaming mountain restaurant. Keep your chin up while being photographed, as the light usually looks more flattering if it hits your face from above – dark circles disappear and double chins melt. A black-and-white photograph is always better than colour.

♥

Don't be tempted to take your photograph at the airport before you jump on the plane. Most skiing holiday packages leave at hideously early times (checking in at 5 a.m. is not unusual), so you will probably feel rushed and may not look your best.

packing your beauty kit

Instead of learning about front-loading ski boots or the latest soon-to-go-out-of-fashion ski wear, focus on beauty equipment. Remember that harsh weather conditions and strenuous exercise affects health as well as beauty, so pack accordingly.

- Shampoo and a rich protein conditioner.
- Bath oil or bubble bath, because one of the best things about skiing is having a heavenly bath afterwards.
- Aspirin for headaches and sunburn.
- Cold/flu remedies.
- Muscle cream.
- Plasters for uncomfortable boots.
- Large pot of dermatological cream.
- Foot cream, particularly those containing peppermint oil or menthol.
- Nail file and clippers for torn or split nails and to keep toenails short for comfort and dancing.
- Petroleum jelly to protect against wind, snow and sleet (but not sun), and for soothing dry patches of skin.

departure beauty

This is your opportunity to shine – not literally but in a gloriously effortless way. Begin the night before by preparing your skin for an inevitably ugly early-morning start. Smooth your face as efficiently as possible, using either a gentle facial exfoliant or by rubbing your face with a slightly damp, warm flannel. Blasting your face with ice, snow, wind and mountain sun in the days to come is assault enough, and this little exercise will ensure that your face looks as radiant and healthy as possible at the start of the holiday. It is also a good idea to treat your hair to a deep conditioning treatment before you go with an extra-rich protein conditioner or hot oil. Like your face, your hair will be subject to the harsh elements and this ensures that it is in peak condition and better able to withstand their detrimental effects.

Do not load your face with make-up for the journey. Heavy make-up never fooled anyone, and when you are tired it makes you look worse and it may make your fellow travellers feel physically sick. Staring at women wearing heavy make-up on the London Underground one morning repulsed an uncle of mine so much that he cut his losses and drove to work instead from then on.

If you cannot bear the thought of turning up naked-faced, wear an extremely light foundation dabbed on the areas where you want some coverage, then brush on a subtle bronzer. Lipstick will make you look like you have tried too hard. Choose a shiny lip balm that will protect your lips on a short but very dehydrating flight.

Unless you are exceptionally nervous and know you suffer from chronic body odour, under no circumstances wear scent or heavily perfumed deodorant. The human nose has evolved to smell out delicious food and recognize our parents and loved ones, not to contend with aggressively smelly molecules. Too much fragrance will just put other travellers off. You will get a bit sweaty and tired in the airport, but this is best dealt with by a citrussy eau de toilette or deodorant stick.

skiing make-up

Ordinary make-up is not a good choice for winter sporting adventures. You will rub off any foundation when you start applying your sunblock anyway. Wearing lipstick and eye make-up on ski slopes always looks a bit like you have been taking tips from Florida housewives. Hopefully, beautifully dyed eyelashes will suffice, but if you have some serious blotches, spots or burst veins to cover, use a waterproof concealer (there are some good ones formulated to cover scar tissue). If you feel unconfident about venturing out without some kind of foundation, moisturize your skin before breakfast, follow with a high-factor sunblock and then add a light helping of foundation or concealer. Finish with a little bronzer or powder, if desired. The pigments in bronzer will provide a tiny bit of extra protection against ultraviolet light because they are made of titanium dioxide.

If gothic eyeliner is part of your raison d'être you are pretty unlikely to be on anything as hearty as a skiing holiday. However, if you cannot bear to be without some sort of eye 'mission statement', choose some vicious-looking sunglasses instead.

The one cosmetic concession that can be worn easily on a skiing holiday is a long-lasting lipstick. Even though the moisture film might disappear, you will be left with a stain of colour that can be freshened up with clear lip block. Some of the latest formulas include antioxidants, which help protect your lips from damage. Choose the most natural colours, such as pinky browns. Alternatively use a lip pencil to colour lips, then slick on lip block, but never take the pencil on the slopes – you do not want to impale yourself if you fall.

ski skincare tips

- ❤ DON'T use astringent or deep-cleansing face packs, especially clay, during a skiing holiday or you will dehydrate skin that is already deprived of moisture.
- ❤ DO drink as much mineral water as you can because altitude is dehydrating – your urine should be straw-coloured or lighter.
- ❤ DON'T drink hot wine during the day if you have high colouring: you will compound the problem.
- ❤ DO use more sunblock than you think you need.
- ❤ DO reapply sunblock at lunchtime. Trying to apply cream on chair lifts is never that successful.
- ❤ DO cover your hairline and ears properly with sunblock.

layer your skin

Protect your skin effectively by layering it with creams in the same way as you dress yourself in layers of clothes to go out on a cold mountain. Bear in mind that when cosmetics companies test their products for SPF protection, they apply quite a thick layer of cream on the skin, so do not be afraid to slather on your sunblock generously and keep reapplying it.

1. First apply a protective antioxidant cream or moisturizer on the face (rather like thermals keeping you cosy under a ski jacket).

2. Layer an SPF25 sunblock on top of the moisturizer.

3. Reapply sunblock every two hours. With increased sweat, falling snow and the dehydrating effects of the strong sunshine, topping up your protective barrier more often will do no harm.

pocket supplies

Have the following products in your pocket on the slopes at all times.

- High-factor ski sunblock.
- Combined lip and eye block.
- Tissues for clearing a cold-air-induced runny nose: frozen crystals around the nostrils are not sexy.
- Emergency loo paper.
- Cold-sore cream.

accident and emergency beauty

However carefully you ski, there is always the risk of an accident and you need to prepare for this. When I fell over and ripped all my knee ligaments I was completely unprepared for what was to follow. Riding in a blood wagon was surprisingly glamorous, swishing over the snow faster than I ever imagined. However, displaying dull, grey and hairy legs to a young, handsome surgeon was not so good. The big tip for skiing is that even if you think you will be swathed in anoraks from dawn until dusk, you cannot always bank on it, so depilation and moisturization give you a little more self-respect.

If you have weak knees, or have previously had a skiing accident, be sure that your legs have enough support. Leg support tubes are available at resort pharmacies and tend to be sturdier than the bandage variety you find in the UK. Contact a doctor if any injury is giving you cause for concern.

Never ski without wearing proper skiing sunglasses or goggles. The strong glare from the snow can damage your eyes. The only time you should take your glasses off is when the light is dull and you feel safer and can see better without them.

Never ski off-piste unless you are with a guide or are an extremely experienced skier. Aside from the potential danger you could be subjecting yourself to, if you are injured off-piste, start an avalanche or inconvenience emergency services, you could be taken to court for causing damages.

Being properly insured is essential. Skiing accidents can be unbelievably expensive and European doctors, especially the Swiss, have a reputation for operating on injuries in the twinkling of an eye, which bumps up bills even more. Carry a credit card with you each day while skiing, in case you need it to guarantee that a blood wagon will be paid – some may refuse to take you unless there is a credit card available.

Bear in mind your natural adrenaline rush if you are unlucky enough to have an accident. People who have a reasonably serious skiing accident often report that they believe – and can – ski or walk for a few minutes after the fall. Do not try to be brave – if the injury is more serious than you realize, you may cause more harm, and anyway, people love rescuing damsels in distress.

Also, do not despair over minor cuts and grazes. A raw chin has a certain glamour and should not be concealed under make-up. Always remember that people love hearing about exotic accidents, so if you should happen to pretend that your graze was caused by an off-piste tumble during an afternoon spent with an Olympic skiing champion, and not from skidding on the wet bathroom floor and cutting your chin on the loo seat, no-one will dare to question you.

how to look like a pro

- ❤ DON'T polish your skis ostentatiously in your chalet each evening.
- ❤ DON'T wear goggles unless it is snowing; wear your sunglasses instead.
- ❤ DON'T wear colourful stripes of zinc block on your face like a tribal leader: this look went out in the 1980s.
- ❤ DON'T wear such a thick layer of total block over your face that you look like a ghost.
- ❤ DO wear a sheer high-protection factor sunblock at all times.
- ❤ DON'T wear high-heeled shoes or boots to totter around the resort – opt for a chunky pair of lace-ups instead.
- ❤ DO chew chewing gum to keep yourself calm and fresh of breath.
- ❤ DON'T wear gaiters to give the impression that you have been skiing off-piste.
- ❤ DON'T publicly try snowboarding if you have never done it before. You will spend 80 per cent of the day on your bottom, so practise it in private first.
- ❤ DO use your ski block as a romantic tool – apply your lip shield alluringly and offer it only to the object of your desire.
- ❤ DON'T take make-up with you on the slopes: what could be more humiliating than being impaled by a lip pencil when you fall over on a mogul?

hair disaster avoidance

Unless you have a few Parisian genes in your make-up, your hair will probably be a disaster on the slopes. I am always amazed how Brits seems to look as if they have had a trainee hairdresser's version of a root perm. Skiing with loose hair is fantastic when you are whistling (momentarily confidently) down a red run, but when it comes to a steep mogul field when you have to concentrate, it is nothing but a hindrance.

Make your first day a trial run and keep a hat in your pocket; if hair starts to look terrible, simply wear your hat. If hair is short, you have few worries. If frizziness is a problem, use slightly more hair serum than usual. If your hair is flyaway, use a little hair serum to flatten the rogue hairs or spritz some hair spray on a comb and gently drag it through your hair. If you do not have hair spray, rub some moisturizer, such as hand cream, in your hands and smooth down your hair. Wear fine, naturally limp hair away from the face, unless you are snowboarding, in which case you will want to look as cerebrally challenged as possible. Whatever your hair type, keep moisture levels high by using a rich conditioner. A common mistake is thinking that overwashing your hair is bad. Top trichologists recommend daily washing and moisturizing of hair to keep it healthy.

Take a few styling tips from the incredibly humourless French women who always look fabulous on skiing holidays. Make sure you have a good cut, then grip hair off and away from the face. As the day progresses, hair will become increasingly sweaty and greasy, but provided it is clipped into place, you will have an appearance of control. Do not, whatever you do, wear hair spray. Snow, ice and water will make most formulas stick and you will end up with truly matted hair.

après-ski beauty

You have stumbled back to the hotel or chalet and you are feeling as glamorous as a Russian shot-putter. Skin is congealed in the day's perspiration, limbs are so tired you can hardly get your boots off. You stagger back to your room only to find someone is in the bathroom. Wrap up warmly so your muscles do not stiffen up, wait your turn and dream of emerging as an après-ski beauty.

When the opportunity arises, run a hot bath, dropping in bath gel, muscle soak or aromatherapy oils. Lavender is a great calmer and perfect for preparing you for the thrill and excitement of jiggling the night away on a hormone-drenched dance floor. If you are feeling exhausted, citrus oils, particularly lemon and grapefruit, are great pick-me-ups. Try to stay in the bath for 20 minutes. Feet always take a bashing during a day's skiing and although a hot bath will not get the swelling down, it will help them relax. Deep breathing will also help you relax more effectively (see page 13). Once out of the bath, wrap up warmly in plenty of towels and a warm dressing-gown. Any draughts or chills will make tired muscles contract and stiffen.

Unless you have been skiing in a bikini, your body will feel a little tired but the skin on your face will really be the problem. However greasy your skin, cleansing should be gentle. If your skin is normal to dry, avoid any vaguely astringent or alkaline (ordinary soap) cleanser. However vigilant you may have been about slathering on protective creams, skin will be dehydrated. To keep water levels high, wash with a moisturizing cleansing cream or bar and cover your face immediately in a thick layer of dermatological cream. Leave the cream on like a face pack while you attend to the rest of your beauty regime. If your skin is naturally dry, by the time you have finished perfuming and slathering on body and muscle cream, your face will have drunk up the whole face pack. Apply a thin layer of eye cream around the eye area. Do not use eye gel on tired, sore eyes because it will not be moisturizing enough.

If your muscles or ligaments are in any pain, and there is a clear difference between an aching, tired muscle and serious mechanical problems, you must not ski or attempt any home-made bandage-wrapping techniques in the hope that everything will be fine. See a doctor or the ski clinic immediately. You could cause serious damage if you ski when even slightly injured. Generally tired but nicely bathed and warmed, muscles in the feet, arms and legs can be massaged back to life easily. Then get into some loose-fitting warm clothes and prepare for a night of après-ski.

foot massage

1. Pour some peppermint or menthol foot lotion onto your hands.

2. Massage your feet by working firmly with your fingers and thumbs over each foot, rubbing from the toes up and along the soles of the feet.

3. Finish by putting on a thick, warm pair of socks. Slippers are far too unsexy and not enveloping enough.

leg and arm massage

1. Massage sports rub into and slightly beyond any problem areas. Do not use too much because the full effect will reach a crescendo of warming a few minutes after application.

2. Use a simple body moisturizer, or something swanky if that is your style, to massage your legs. Start at the feet or ankles and move up towards the hips.

3. Use the moisturizer to massage your arms, working from your hands up.

saunas and steams

Saunas, however heavenly an idea at the end of a hard day's exercise, put the capillaries in the skin under enormous pressure. Just as you have escaped the elements and extreme changes of temperature during the day, the blood vessels in your face will not know what has hit them. If you think you are going to miss out on a fabulous opportunity to relax or compare cellulite quantities and beer belly sizes with your skiing party, suggest a steam room over a sauna. The moist heat will be better for your skin than dry sauna heat and you can appear as a fetching mirage through the clouds of steam.

nightlife

Something very strange seems to happen to people's energy levels on skiing holidays. However physically exhausted you may be by late afternoon after a day on the slopes, at night-time you come alive again. Theories on why this happens abound. Some put it down to high spirits, love interests or adrenaline highs after a day of exhilaration and fear, but the most likely theory seems to be oxygen deprivation. The human body apparently functions better in 15 per cent oxygen – ordinary air contains 21 per cent. The result is higher energy levels and a heightened sense of wellbeing.

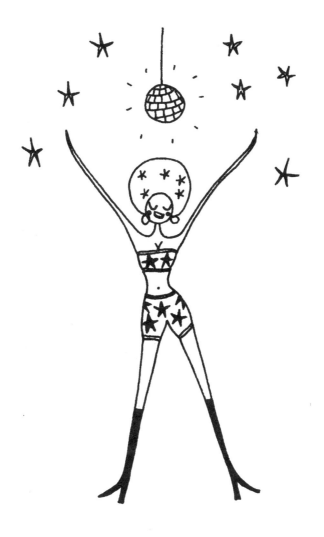

Nightlife in ski resorts is not the most sophisticated way to pass time. Unless you are staying in a super luxury hotel complete with shaggy rugs and crackling log fires, the chances are you will be frequenting bars, restaurants and nightclubs surrounded by people with bright red faces and hearty laughs. Looking like a natural beauty when you are puce in the face and covered in sweat on an Alpine dance floor requires a little effort. Although having matted hair and punching the air to the time of a recent chart hit is sadly unavoidable, having make-up running down your face while you are participating in this pastime is. For a smear-proof party look, follow the tips listed below.

disco diva make-up tips

- ❤ DO wear waterproof make-up, particularly mascara.
- ❤ DO use oil-free or oil-absorbing tinted moisturizer for a healthy but not shiny glow.
- ❤ DON'T wear any foundation at all – it will just make you look grey.
- ❤ DON'T wear a green colour-correction foundation to counteract redness – it will look dreadful and fake.
- ❤ DON'T wear a lurid shade of lipstick. However fabulous it looks when you swirl around parties at home, on a rosy-red face, it will clash.
- ❤ DO wear a slightly shimmery lip gloss for a prettier and more natural look.

next day recovery plan

A morning ski face is something rather unique. Satisfyingly, even some of the most ravishing among us suffer the same après après-ski face as us ordinary mortals. Thanks to the high altitude, sweating on a dance floor or the equatorial humidity level in a horribly jolly fondue restaurant, the skin on the face is parched. Eyes are extraordinarily puffy – puffier than you have ever known – and lips are dry and flaking.

The dehydrated face is easily remedied. Simply splash your face with cool to tepid water (which will help deflate any puffiness a little), then slather on a rich moisturizer. Follow with a good sunblock to prepare the skin for another day of assault.

A slick of a good lip salve or petroleum jelly will help flaking lips. As someone who has suffered from more than my share of Parmesan lips, I do not adhere to the method of exfoliating lips with an old toothbrush. Exfoliation just rubs off even more bits of dried skin and makes lips look worse. The best advice I have been given was from a down-to-earth dermatologist who recommended applying lip salve regularly, every few minutes if necessary, to help give the lips a chance to recover their own moisture levels.

Eyes require a philosophical approach rather than hoping for a miracle. Bags will deflate as the morning progresses and even blinking will help disperse the puffiness. A little eye gel gives a refreshing sensation and may help reduce bags faster. Apply by using your ring finger to 'tap' the gel over the entire eye-socket area. If your eyelids feel a little sore and dry, only treat the under-eye area. For a desperate measure, scoop up a handful of freshly fallen snow from the windowsill. Arrange the snow in a 5-cm (2-inch) thick line along the length of a face flannel. Fold the flannel in half and lay it across your eyes. Do not put snow directly on your eyes as it could be too harsh for your skin. Leave the flannel on your eyes until it no longer feels cold. Remember to put a towel under your head to catch drips of melting snow.

post-ski maintenance

Depending on your ration of toxic consumption, late nights and healthy days spent inhaling mountain air, you will return from the skiing trip either looking dreadful – albeit sunkissed – or glowing with health and hale and hearty.

Unless you are lucky enough to have extremely dark skin, you will most likely be sporting 'panda eyes', thanks to your goggles. Do not try to fill in the white areas with fake tan. Instead, mix a little tinted mosturizer with foundation and apply it in tiny dots around the eye socket, blending it outwards. A light dusting of bronzer under the eyes will also give you a uniform colour, but do not use too much or the powder will cause lines to appear.

Tanned skin is damaged skin and your dermis will be draining its resources trying to repair itself. For the next few days after you get back, moisturize obsessively and drink lots of water to revitalize your dehydrated skin and restore a healthy, dewy look.

chapter four

the toxic weekend

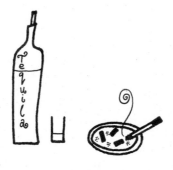

Most of us learn about toxic weekends early in life. The combination of chain-smoking Russian cigarettes and dancing creatively to Abba has little or no effect in our teenage years. Then one day, sometime in our twenties, it happens. You wake up after a late alcohol-drenched night and find the Gorgon glaring back from the mirror. Inky-black rings encircle your eyes, the bags under them look as if you have experimented with a DIY collagen kit and your complexion has turned to putty. I would be lying if I said that all of this can be avoided, but you can go a long way to tone down the nightmarish spectre. There is, of course, a certain glamour in being utterly revolting for a limited period of time, but it is unnecessary. And there is nothing more smug-making than feeling better than you really should.

Lethargy and hangovers can be eased or even eradicated by avoiding certain foods and resisting cravings. Clever cosmetic masks can work wonders to perk up toxic-looking skin, and using the right combination of skincare and make-up also has a miraculous effect in transforming a frighteningly unhealthy pallor into one of peachy perfection.

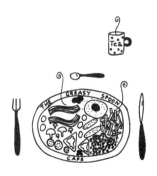

night repair

Night creams, applied before you collapse into bed after an evening of indulgence, will help leave you more fresh-faced in the morning. The skin repairs itself at night, ready to protect and defend against the elements the following day. According to experts, the body repairs at the optimum level between the hours of 11 p.m. and 3 a.m. In fact, the body is so responsive at this time that certain drugs cannot be administered at night because they are too quickly absorbed – they have to be given during the day when the body is more 'distracted'.

Most day creams now contain sunscreens, which are not needed when you are asleep, so buy a cream specifically formulated for night use, preferably one that claims to boost skin circulation or which contains antioxidants (see pages 212 and 240). Some simple night cream formulas are just heavy moisturizers. Visit a cosmetics counter and ask about their most recent formulas. Because the cosmetics market is so competitive, companies have to update their formulas regularly to keep other brands from swiping their share of the market.

retinol and antioxidant creams

'Nourishing' as well as moisturizing skin is becoming a big issue in skincare and can make all the difference to a toxic-

or not-so-toxic-looking face. Basically, moisturizing just keeps water in the skin, but skin food, such as antioxidants and vitamins, helps improve the ability of the skin to function. Some of the newest creams contain retinol, a vitamin A derivative (see pages 214 and 246), which works most effectively away from ultraviolet light. The benefits of retinol include increased cell renewal and improved collagen and elastin building, resulting in firmer, brighter-looking skin. Other night-time workers are antioxidants, such as vitamins E and C and extracts of grapeseed and green tea, which help the skin recover after a night of smoke and other pollutants. Vitamin C is a particularly good rejuvenator but is very unstable. Because it can only remain active – and so effective – for a short time once exposed to air, it is often packaged in phials which you have to mix together to use. More recently, cosmetics companies have encapsulated vitamin C in microbubbles, which keep the vitamin airtight and fresh. The micro-bubbles are too small to see in a cream but once applied, they enter the layers of the skin, the bubbles break down naturally and the vitamin is released. Vitamins E and A are also available in this microbubble delivery system.

If you want to give your skin the equivalent of a neat vodka shot rather than a vodka and tonic, use a serum. These will not moisturize the skin, but they will gorge your skin on vitamins or anti-ageing ingredients. Apply a serum, letting the skin soak it up, then add a moisturizer on top.

oxygen creams

Another good night-time choice is an oxygen cream. They work on the principle that oxygen molecules are delivered into the skin via the cream, circulation then improves and cells work harder and repair more enthusiastically. Some oxygen creams are mixed with other skin-beautifying ingredients, so choose one that offers the best combination for you. If, for example, your skin tends to be a little dull and grey, try an oxygen and AHA (see page 240) combination, which will help smooth the skin and slough off dead cells.

essential oil formulas

An alternative to a night cream is using a prepared essential oil formulated for the face. The molecules of essential oil penetrate deeper into the skin than many other cosmetic ingredients. The oil improves skin circulation, resulting in brighter, more radiant skin. You must use a ready-blended formula. Never apply neat essential oil to the skin because it is far too strong and likely to cause irritation. Do not confuse proper essential oil preparations with token 'aromatherapy' products, which may have a minute amount of essential oil included. Good-quality essential oil products have to be stored in dark glass bottles or jars because plastic does not protect the oil effectively.

night-time repair solutions

- For a basic recovery, use creams that include vitamin E and general antioxidant 'cocktails'.
- For recovery plus radiance, use formulas that contain vitamin C and oxygen.
- For turbo-charging skin firmness, choose retinol creams to repair collagen and elastin.
- For a healthy bloom, use an oxygen cream.
- To combat dull, grey skin, choose an AHA or BHA cream that contains salicylic acid, fruit acid or glycolic acid (see pages 218–19).

prepare ahead

If you plan to throw caution to the wind and indulge in a weekend of late, alcohol-drenched and smoke-fumed nights, there are a few preparation steps you can take to help you go the distance. Daytime hours during the weekend will probably be spent trying to regain some sense of normality – even if only to destroy it again the following evening.

Stocking up on nutritional and skincare treats will go a long way towards remedying a body and beauty hangover the next day, but there are also steps you can take to protect your skin against clouds of cigarette smoke and to look good all night long.

stocking up for recovery

♥ DO stock your fridge with lots of mineral water and alkaline fruit drink to help neutralize the acidity caused by alcohol.

♥ DO buy a melon, a selection of citrus fruit, beans, pulses and fresh vegetables you like eating (there is no point in being too self-sacrificing). All are helpful toxic antidotes.

♥ DON'T buy ready-made fruit juice unless it is preservative-free.

♥ DON'T buy frozen ready-meals or the ingredients for a fry-up breakfast. If they are not available, you will not be tempted.

♥ DO place a wet flannel in a polythene bag and keep it in the fridge for placing over your eyes the next morning. Alternatively, buy a gel-filled eye mask.

♥ DO have a supply of night cream, eye gel, headache tablets and vitamin C.

face the party

♥ Use an anti-pollutant moisturizer that boasts anti-oxidants and an SPF15 or more.

♥ Wear a foundation with similar ingredients as well as moisturizers to help protect your skin against smoke and dehydration.

💗 If you want to keep looking flawless for as long as possible, wear a long-lasting foundation that should withstand even the most marathon dance session.

💗 If you tend to look washed out by the early hours, apply a little fake tan before you go out (see page 31). By the time all the other lovelies are wilting, you will look as fresh as a daisy.

bedtime routine

When you do get back in the early hours, force yourself to follow these simple steps.

1. Remove all your make-up.

2. Apply a night cream or serum.

3. Apply an eye cream formulated for bedtime use.

4. Drink a pint of water.

5. Pop a vitamin C supplement to help kick-start the body's recovery process.

6. Provided you are not too away with the fairies, apply some fake tan (see page 31). You will wake up looking one thousand times healthier than you would otherwise.

morning-after eyes

Eyes give the game away on lack of sleep. The world seems to divide into puffy-eyed and dark-circle victims. A classic mistake many people make is applying moisturizer, especially rich, heavy formulas, all over the face including the eye area. The skin around the eyes is extremely thin and becomes overwhelmed by heavy face cream, which causes puffiness. If you do not have an eye cream or gel and puffiness is a problem, avoid putting any moisturizer under the eye altogether. Although baby oil is a good, cheap eye make-up remover, it may make eyes puffy because it can be too heavy. If you do use baby oil, make sure you wipe it off thoroughly with cotton wool.

Dark circles are harder to treat, and are caused by poor circulation, dehydration and lack of sleep. Drinking a pint of water before bed will help, but learning how to put on

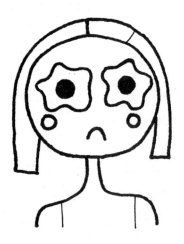

under-eye concealer is a more realistic solution. Some new eye creams claim to reduce or 'diminish' dark circles, and they do seem to work a little. In order to claim that a cream treats dark circles, the dark circles do not have to disappear but just have to be slightly reduced. The most effective formulas tend to contain a tiny helping of light-diffusing particles or even a little pigment which masks the intensity of the rings.

Good ingredients to look for in before-bed eye creams include fish cartilage extract, vitamin K and classic beauty ingredients such as witch hazel. Eye gels are better used as bag deflators the following morning.

eye bag remover warning

Haemorrhoid-treatment cream is a well-known eye-bag deflator and is often used by make-up artists – even the odd celebrity admits to it. Using this cream, however, is really a desperate measure, undignified and unnecessary. Bags are never that bad for long and there are plenty of famous beauties like Greta Scaatchi who look fabulous with baggy eyes. Also, try telling your new amour that you are actually using haemorrhoid cream to reduce the bags under your eyes and he will probably pass out in disgust, whether he believes you or not.

morning-after skincare

If your skin looks grey and pasty the morning after a night of indulgence, start by sloughing off the surface layer of dead skin cells and improving the circulation in the skin. If you tend towards oiliness rather than dryness, use a gentle exfoliating cream that includes salicylic acid or AHAs. Because the complexion-dulling old cells are being shed faster than usual, younger, fresher and ultimately more radiant cells are encouraged to renew at a quicker rate. Enzyme moisturizers (see page 219) work along similar lines, but because they simply loosen the intercellular cement, or 'glue', that holds cells together, they are a gentler option and the best choice for drier skins. If you do not have an exfoliant, a clean flannel or a piece of muslin massaged gently over the face will do a similar job, but probably will not leave your skin feeling quite as silky as a face exfoliant. In addition to improving your complexion, a face scrub will also help refresh and revive a tired face.

Follow the scrub with an intensive moisturizing mask or layer on your daily moisturizer thickly, leaving it to soak in. Alternatively, try a home-made mask (see opposite). Do not use a clay or astringent mask because these are drying, and you need to keep as much natural moisture in the skin as possible. Clay dries on the face, drawing out grease and other impurities, but also moisture.

refreshing yoghurt face mask

The fruit and lactic acid in the mask will help smooth skin, and you can eat the remaining mixture for breakfast to help beat your hangover.

1. Mix some natural yoghurt and lime juice together.

2. Apply the mixture as a face mask, spreading it on thickly, and leave it for 10 minutes to work on your skin.

3. Rinse the mixture off thoroughly with warm water.

4. Pat your face dry and apply a moisturizer.

egg-white face mask

The egg white has a tightening effect and is best for combination or oily skins.

1. Beat together an egg white and the juice of half a lemon.

2. Spread the mask on thickly and leave it for 10 minutes.

3. Rinse it off thoroughly with warm water.

4. Pat your face dry and apply moisturizer.

easy face revivers

♥ After washing or cleansing your face, take a chilled, damp flannel from the fridge and place it over your face, pressing it gently into the contours. When the flannel no longer feels cold, remove it and pat your face dry. This will help you wake up, reduce puffiness and raise colour in the cheeks.

♥ If you are still feeling dopey, squeeze your ears quite firmly between your entire thumb and index finder. This Oriental massage technique has an extraordinarily rapid reviving effect.

♥ Try a pressure-point massage. Press the inner eyebrows with your index fingers, then keep pressing along the line of your brows until you reach your temples. Then work your fingers around the top of your cheekbones, moving inwards towards the gum line of the upper jaw.

♥ If you have no beauty products to hand, and your eyes are very puffy and your skin looks grey, splash your face repeatedly with very cold water and then pat it dry with a towel.

♥ To give your skin even more of a boost, use a face pack that claims to be rejuvenating. Anything that contains menthol or eucalyptus will feel refreshing on the skin, but avoid face packs that contain these ingredients if your skin is sensitive or dry.

body reviver

Trick your skin into feeling revived by dry body brushing (see pages 20–1). Because of its supposed detoxifying effects, body brushing could also be considered a valiant attempt to help skin expel some of the toxins that you have treated it to.

1. Using short, firm strokes, brush from the hands along the arms towards your heart.

2. Brush from the soles of the feet to the tops of the legs.

3. Follow with a warm, but not hot, shower to continue the zombie revival programme.

morning exercise

A drained, white complexion can be improved in minutes with a little gentle exercise. Although you might not be in the state of mind for strenuous activity, yoga exercises are enlivening. One of the best is a stretch called the 'Down Dog'. An important posture in yoga, it stretches legs, back, arms and shoulders and gets blood to your head to restore a healthy glow. The exercise will help stretch out any tight muscles you may have from trying Elvis Presley impersonations on the dance floor the night before. The Triangle posture also has a surprisingly reviving effect.

down dog

1. Stand with your feet flat on the floor, about 30 cm (1 foot) apart.

2. Bend forward, bending your knees, until your hands are flat on the floor, parallel to each other with your fingers spread as widely as is comfortable.

3. Let your head hang down and straighten your arms, keeping your knees bent.

4. When your arms are supporting half your body weight, start straightening your legs. Your heels will naturally lift off the floor.

5. Push your bottom up to the ceiling and your heels down, with your hands flat on the floor.

6. Hold the position, enjoying the stretch.

7. For best results, breathe in deeply and noisily through the nose and out again through slightly pursed lips for 10 breaths.

8. Gently walk your hands back towards your feet and slowly uncurl you body into an upright position.

the triangle

1. Begin by standing with your feet about 90 cm (3 feet) apart, facing forward. Point your left toe in, towards your right leg.

2. Move your right foot 45 degrees out, so your toes are pointing away from their starting position.

3. Raise your arms straight out to the sides, parallel to the floor, with palms facing down and fingers outstretched.

4. Bend sideways to the right, keeping your arms straight, until your right hand touches your right shin. Keep your legs straight.

5. Your left arm should be pointing to the ceiling. Turn the palm out to face ahead and look up towards it, focusing on your thumb.

6. Hold the position and breathe deeply (see step 7 of Down Dog, opposite) for five deep breaths.

7. Slowly and gently uncurl your body and return to the starting position.

8. Repeat the exercise on the other side of the body.

detoxifying baths

Our European neighbours are much better than we Anglo-Saxons at smoking, eating and drinking themselves into oblivion and then purging themselves with detoxifying treatments. I will never forget my experience in a Moroccan hammam in a hot and sweaty corner of the country one summer. A gang of huge Moroccan women, clad only in industrial-sized black knickers, stared at my comparatively scrawny frame. I found a friend of mine in the massage room lying flat on the floor having her back massaged by a large Moroccan foot. Of course you do not have to go to the drastic measures of plunging yourself in alternating freezing cold and boiling hot water, but a soak in a detoxifying bath might ease an otherwise exhausted body back to a little more life.

You can help your body dispel poisons by body brushing (see pages 20–1 and 119) followed by a bath. Because marine extracts are well known for their detoxifying effects, buy sachets of sea algae soaks to add to a warm bath. If you cannot face wallowing around hippo-style in a smelly algae bath, then sea-salt soaks are a good alternative. Be wary of marine ingredients if you suspect your skin is sensitive to them.

If you are severely hung-over, the prospect of a smelly algae bath could make you feel worse. In this case, a better choice would be to add four to five drops of an essential oil to the bath. Good detoxifying oils include rosemary, citrus oils and juniper. For a really exotic experience, scent the air around you using an essential oil burner or candles.

Abdominal breathing in the bath will help your hung-over body detoxify faster too. Beauty therapists sometimes ask their clients to do a little deep breathing, not only to relax them but also to inhale the aroma of the oils and boost oxygen levels in the body. Simply breathe deeply, concentrating on filling your stomach – imagine filling your lower stomach with air rather than your chest. Check that you are breathing effectively by placing a hand on your stomach and watching it swell. Your shoulders should not rise as you inhale; if they do, you are not breathing correctly. The stomach should inflate as you inhale and deflate as you exhale.

eat away your hangover

The best antidote to a late, toxic night, apart from cleverly applied make-up, is eating well the next day. Most of us crave a fantastically unhealthy breakfast after a night of overindulgence. Sugar-coated cereal always tastes delicious when you are tired and for some reason even aspiring vegans abandon their principles and sink their chops into everything from black pudding to fried bread. The reason most of us are desperate for this sort of food is

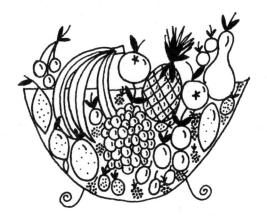

straightforward: simple sugars give an immediate sense of energy. Unlike the more complex forms of sugar found in fresh vegetables, simple sugars are extremely easy for the body to absorb and process and give you a shot of energy. However, this sugar 'high' is not sustaining, so a little later, you experience a 'low' when blood sugar levels drop. Combine sugar with wheat and dairy products that make you sluggish and you have a recipe for lethargy and light-headedness.

Some nutritionists argue that the overconsumption of fats and salt, which are found in meat and processed food, encourage the excessive consumption of cold drinks, and the chances are that you will reach for sugary fizzy drinks that do nothing to help the body rebalance. The best thing you can do is reach for the mineral water. Try to drink as much water as you can to help your body flush out the toxins and rehydrate itself.

liver-loving pick-me-ups

If your hangover is bad, your liver will be working overtime, sifting nasty toxins out. Eat food that provides long-lasting energy and drink home-made fruit juice to help provide healthy, energizing sugars. Melon juice is one of the best antidotes to a tired, toxic body. Unlike some citrus fruits, such as orange and grapefruit, melon is gentle on the stomach, yet contains plenty of nourishment. Aloe vera juice, found in good health food shops, is another excellent liver-function support drink. If you do not have any fruit juice, vitamin C supplements should help. Vitamin C will help counter the effects of smoking (which kills off vitamin C in the body) and bolster your immune system for further onslaughts of late nights and unhealthy eating.

toxic weekend food guidelines

- ❤ DO start the day with some fruit juice, and bananas for energy.
- ❤ DO eat muesli. Muesli takes longer to digest, so provides the body with more 'fuel' to clear out toxins from the night before.
- ❤ DON'T drink sweet, carbonated drinks, even if they are diet drinks.
- ❤ DO drink still water. Ideally it should be mineral or filtered, but if necessary, just drink good old tap.

- DO drink fruit juice, especially melon or aloe vera.
- DON'T try to wake yourself up with coffee.
- DO drink tea: it still contains caffeine but will not be as brutal.
- DON'T eat sugary breakfast cereals, greasy fry-ups or tempting burgers and chips. You will only feel worse for longer if you do.

reviving food

Leslie Kenton, the ground-breaking author of numerous books on health and beauty, is well known for her belief in 'raw energy'. Eating raw, organic food helps boost the immune system and is a superior fuel for the body. To help your body feel more energetic, try not to mix proteins and carbohydrates at the same meal, which can make you feel sluggish. Fruit juice can help combat a hangover and, according to Kenton, carrot and apple juice are a good combination.

If you are feeling sluggish and low after your toxic whirl, give your body a break and a boost by following a careful diet for three days. The bottom line is to cut out all dairy and wheat products, apart from milk in tea or coffee. Also drink two litres of still mineral water each day, and no more than two cups of tea or coffee. A couple of glasses of fruit juice a day is plenty – too much is likely to upset a delicate stomach.

detox diet

For breakfast: Eat only fruit, but avoid excessive quantities of citrus fruit, including pineapple. Bananas, apples, melon and pears are all excellent choices. If you want something more filling, eat authentic rye bread (make sure it is wheat-free) and honey.

For lunch and supper: Eat anything you like, provided it is healthy and fresh, but avoid dairy or wheat products. Pasta, pizzas and yoghurt are out. Do not eat diet food: some are formulated to expand in your stomach and can cause bloating.

suddenly sensitive

Late nights, incalculable helpings of alcohol, general showing off or even stressful social situations can provoke the odd allergy or rash. Red wine can bring out terrible blotches in some people. If skin feels very tender and you cannot face washing or cleansing it with your normal skincare products, use an emulsifying cream. Basically a simple blend of oil and water, the cream can be used to remove make-up and moisturize. Although there are a number of extremely good dermatological creams on the market, sold to help soothe contact dermatitis, rashes or detergent hands, for example, I have found that they do not really help an irritated face. If anything, they are too rich, making the skin feel suffocated, yet strangely dehydrated. Emulsifying cream, which can be mixed up for you by a chemist, is better, if a little greasy-looking. Apply it in a thick layer over the face as a moisturizing mask. A good toner for sensitive skin is a mixture of one-third rose-water, one-third distilled water and one-third witch hazel, which you can get from a chemist. Chill the rose-water toner, then pour some onto cotton wool pads and place them over the eyes to deflate bags, or swipe one over the face to refresh the skin.

For any sort of rash, take some antihistamine tablets. This will calm down an already raging immune system. If your rash is still bad the following morning, dab on a little hydrocortisone cream to help contract dilated, overexcited blood vessels and make the rash less visible. A very low-dosage hydrocortisone cream is available over chemists' counters. Do not use it near or on the eyes and only use it on the face if you have discussed this with your doctor.

For tingling, pre-cold sore lips, dab on cold sore treatment cream or neat tea tree oil. Make sure you use authentic tea tree oil from the only variety of tea trees that actually produce the antibacterial, antifungal oil, *Melaleuca alternifolia*. Some people say that holding a slightly dampened soluble aspirin against the sore also helps. Another remedy is to take lysine tablets. Lysine is an amino acid that fights the chemicals that encourage cold sores to develop.

toxic shock make-up

A tired, dull face often looks worse when made up, but the prospect of going out bare-faced is a far more terrifying thought. Because make-up is now so fantastically subtle, you should have no excuse for looking anything but bright-eyed and bushy-tailed.

The golden rule is to avoid caking your face with cosmetics, however desperate you might be feeling. The most important step before putting on any make-up at all is to get your skin smooth and hydrated by using an exfoliator and moisturizing mask (see page 117). Also put some lip balm or petroleum jelly on your lips to plump them up, ready for lipstick or gloss.

Some well-known 'skin perkers' do have a remarkably enlivening effect. A few of the formulas have been around for years and held in highest regard by television personalities and make-up artists alike. Ask at the counter of your favourite brand if they have any 'instant lift' beauty products. They may vary from face masks to fluids that you apply just before make-up.

Although investing in complexion-tinting foundations and what are grandly called 'pre-foundation primers' is tempting, the best way to eradicate a tired face and fake a healthy glow is to apply foundation in very thin layers only where it is most needed.

Other than using a cosmetic sponge, which wastes foundation by absorbing it, the best way to apply foundation is to put a little blob on the back of the hand, near the thumb joint, and slowly build up the layers by blending it with your fingers. Keep make-up natural and clean-looking (see pages 176–8) and follow the tips below for acquiring a fresh glowing look. If your face lets you down, beautifully clean, shiny hair will help distract from your toxic complexion.

fresh look make-up tips

- ❤ DO thicken eyelashes with mascara and shape brows – luckily these features are not in the slightest bit affected by late nights.
- ❤ DO rub some cream blusher directly onto the apples of your cheeks, then apply a little foundation on top. The effect will make you look flushed with health.
- ❤ DO brush a little matte, pink blusher or eyeshadow under your eyes to reduce dark circles.
- ❤ DO brush a little bronzer over your forehead, down your nose and over your chin and cheekbones to give a deceptively healthy look. Choose a very sheer, barely noticeable texture and brush it where the sun naturally hits the face.

- DO use a little lip pencil shaded all over your lips, slicking lip gloss on top.
- DON'T use powder, especially around your eyes, as it can make tired skin look worse.
- DON'T wear eyeshadow on tired eyelids.
- DON'T wear a strong-coloured lipstick: it will destroy the natural effect and look ghoulish.

blood-shot eye antidote

Pink eyes are a give-away. Try some of the measures here to reduce their unfortunate impact.

- Clear pinkness by using eye drops. If you wear contact lenses, check with an optician that the drops are safe to use.
- Avoid brown, pink or purple eyeliner or eyeshadow.
- Use a pale ivory or bluey-white eyeshadow over your eyelids: a blue tone will counteract the red.
- If the skin around your eyes is pink, dot a tiny amount of concealer on the corners of the eyes and blend it in.

new-age action

If the idea of eating nutritious food or slathering on face packs bores you – or does not fit in with the general earthiness of a toxic weekend – some Glastonbury-style therapies might appeal to you more. Top of the list are crystal healing and flower and colour therapies, but the bottom line is that they are all to do with 'vibrations', which is quite appropriate if you have been gyrating to eardrum-bursting music the night before. If you are slightly cynical of things 'touchy-feely', this section will not be for you and you should go and mix yourself a nice face pack and relax. But for any aspiring new-age types, read on.

crystal healing

The basic theory is that crystals have an electro-magnetic energy, which vibrates and can clear any emotional and – many believe – physical blockages in the human body. Because everything in the world is composed of jiggling atoms, the power of the crystal (if you believe it exists) can be used to realign the energy in the body and mind. Crystals can also be used as an aid to meditation and visualization to help focus the mind.

Different crystals can be used to heal a variety of problems. For example, the ancient Chinese used jade to treat bladder and kidney problems. The theory is complex, and crystal therapy cannot just be picked up and tried in the comfort of your own home, but if you are interested in clearing your head, increasing energy and rebalancing your body, the therapy might be worth investigating (see directory, page 253).

colour therapy

This therapy relies on vibrational healing and certain colours are believed to have different effects on the mind and body. In fact, cosmetics companies are now selling scented, coloured bath oils to revive or refresh. If you are feeling really dedicated, or so hung-over that you are unfit for even monosyllabic conversation, you could spend some of the day charging water with the appropriate colour. To do this, pour some water into a coloured glass bottle or place some coloured glass in front of an ordinary clear glass or jar, positioning it so that light from a window shines into the water. Leave it in sunlight for four hours and then drink it.

Ayurvedic, a traditional Indian medicine, places great importance on the healing or disruptive effect of coloured food. If your liver needs some help after a toxic splurge, try eating red foods, such as red cabbage, cherries, cranberry juice and blackberries.

Ayurvedic medicine divides people into three main categories, vata, pitta and kapha, and each one of these can be rebalanced by particular colours. If your main weaknesses are anxiety, fear and overexcitement, you are vata; if your negative sides include anger, frustration, jealousy, hostility and exhaustion, you are pitta; and if you are prone to being be lethargic, depressive and sorry for yourself, you are kapha.

colour codes

Vata: You can be calmed by warm, muted colours and benefit from wearing or looking at gold, orange, yellow, deep purple, indigo and brown. Avoid red.

Pitta: You would benefit from cool colours, such as white, pale blues and greens, and should avoid bright or dark colours.

Kapha: You need bright colours, such as scarlet, orange and yellow. Avoid wishy-washy pink, white, blue and brown.

flower therapy

Although based on the same vibration principles as colour therapy, flower therapy is much easier to explore because you can buy flower essences at even the smallest chemists. According to therapists in this field, different flowers give off specific vibrations and the result of these vibrations can help various physical and emotional problems, from period pain to panic. Different brands of flower remedies use the same flowers to treat slightly varying conditions and problems, but they all work on the same principle.

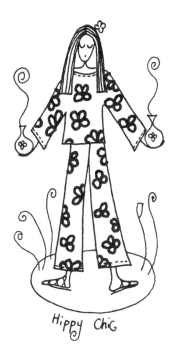

Hippy Chic

The Bach Flower Remedies are some of the most readily available. Dr Edward Bach created his flower-healing system in the 1930s and is widely acknowledged to be the British authority on flower healing. The essences come in little bottles, usually with a rubber pipette dropper. They can either be taken by dropping the liquid under the tongue or mixing it with water or soft drinks, but never dilute them with tea or coffee. Drops can also be added to a bath and you should soak in the water for up to 30 minutes. For sensitive skin conditions, drops can be diluted with pure spring water and splashed on the skin. Alternatively, fill a plant spray container with spring water, add four to six drops of the essence and spray on the skin.

flower power for the partied-out

- For anger (at your dreadful behaviour): holly.
- For bitterness (at the thought of seeing your ex dancing with a beautiful nubile new lovely): willow.
- To calm (you have met Prince Charming and are unlikely to ever see him again): white chestnut.
- For clarity of mind (when giving your friend love advice after the exciting night before): white chestnut.
- For daydreaming (your mind keeps drifting off to your fabulous new-found dancing technique): clematis.
- For fear (at facing all those people again): rock rose.
- For guilt (showing off about a new fictitious beau): pine.

revving up a flagging battery

Clever beauty lotions and make-up techniques are all very well, but when it comes to revving up for a second night of fun, you will need a bit more help to get yourself in the mood and looking as ravishing as usual. A warm bath, containing the right aromatherapy oil, makes a start. Citrus oil is the most reviving and actually tricks the brain into waking up (see also pages 122–3 for a detoxifying bath). Give yourself at least 15 minutes for soaking and relaxing, then set an alarm clock for a 20-minute sleep. You will probably feel groggy on waking, but after about 10 minutes you will feel much more refreshed.

For make-up, employ the tips suggested on page 130. Avoid wearing a heavy foundation or the skin will just look waxy and lifeless. A common mistake is believing that the lower the light, the heavier make-up should be. In reality, the lower the light, the less make-up you are likely to need.

Defining eyes and lips is the most important part of evening make-up. If your eyes look as if they are retreating to the back of your brain, use a dark eyeliner close to the tops of the upper eyelashes, sweeping it down to the outer edges of the lashes. White eyeliner on the inside of the lower lashes freshens up the whites of the eyes. A little eyeshadow highlighter right underneath the eyebrows also wakes the face up and this little trick is less detectable in soft evening light than in daylight.

the final stage

It is Sunday night and you look dreadful and feel completely exhausted. Here are some tips to help you face the start of another new week.

- ❤ Eat comforting and soothing food. All the pulses you stocked up with (a tin of baked beans will do) will give you a protein kick to help ease your body back to life.
- ❤ Drink a pint of water before bed to purge your dehydrated body with cleaning fluid.
- ❤ Tuck up in bed wearing a double helping of moisturizer.

chapter five

the hearty break

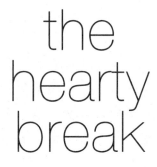

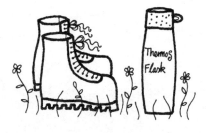

Once the preserve of ornithologists and ramblers, hearty breaks are now becoming surprisingly fashionable. But I am not talking about yomping around shouting 'hurrah' at the tops of your lungs like the Famous Five or carbo-loading in farmers' kitchens. Part of the recent interest in outdoor-oriented breaks is to glow with renewed energy and health, to wear shabby-chic clothes, to have hair blown carelessly by the wind and to have the lust for designer goods blown asunder by the smell of earth and green grass. A hearty break means an entirely unique sort of beauty challenge. In order to preserve the façade of natural beauty you must conceal your efforts with the furtiveness of a suburban transvestite.

Hearty breaks separate the men from the boys, the girls from the girlies. They realign you with the real issues – like the fact that you love make-up and scented baths – and enable you to return looking and feeling genuinely healthy. One friend of mine undergoes a complete personality change on a hearty break. She mutates from London lounge-lizard to Boadicea in walking boots. She swims in icy streams, the temperature of which she would not ordinarily consider rinsing lettuce leaves in, and walks further than the entire London Underground network in one day.

If you are more polluted party girl than a *Country Life* fresh face, or if you are staying with a boyfriend's parents who are disdainful of urban and suburban trimmings, this chapter will be your guide to faking the healthy outdoor look.

be prepared: take a tip from the girl guides

Hearty breakers' disdain for anything synthetic is almost as obsessive as the Dissolution of the Monasteries. However much you love your petrol-coloured nail polish and long talons, clinging to boulders and absailing ropes with them will make you feel foolish and more out of place than you can imagine. You will also be set up as a glamour puss, an almost impossible achievement under such circumstances, and only open to ridicule. The aim is to create an air of charming cool and tremendous natural beauty, no matter what Herculean tasks are set before you or what bodily functions you are aware of. Although this may sound like an impossible feat, all you have to do is plan a week ahead with the precision of an army general.

nail care

Complaining about a broken nail when the general conversation is moving from crampons to resurrecting the peat-burning industry is a brave move. Have a professional manicure and pedicure or set some time aside to do it yourself. Remove all nail polish and file nails down to an elegant but practical length. Rub some oil into your nails to keep their moisture levels high and help prevent unnecessary splits and breaks.

effortless hair

Recently trimmed and conditioned hair will still look good and keep its shape, even when blown in the wind on the top of Snowdon or during a quick Kendal Mint Cake fix behind a boulder with a hearty break hero. A really intensive hydrating treatment the night before you leave will help increase moisture reserves in the hair and protect against the battering from wind, rain or sea spray. Hot oil treatments are good for very dry, wiry or curly hair and lighter hair packs are best for fine, flyaway hair. Alternatively, try a home-made treatment, which you may even be able to sneak in while you are away (see avocado, page 152). A body-building blow dry will last for several days and help you avoid looking like a 1970s folk-singer after an hour's walking. Buy some dry shampoo to take with you. Although almost everyone I know thinks dry shampoo is one of the world's most revolting concepts, it is miraculous stuff that may save the day (see page 150).

eye dye

For a natural look without make-up, dye your eyelashes. You can either have a salon treatment or do it yourself using a kit bought from a chemist, in which case you must remember to spread plenty of petroleum jelly over the skin around the eyes to protect it from the dye. Having your eyebrows professionally shaped, either by plucking or waxing, and dyed makes your face look groomed and tidy. One of the most extraordinary 'bored housewife' inventions is perming the eyelashes. This does have its merits as a curly eyelash 'opens' the eye, making it look bigger and more awake – handy when you emerge from a smelly tent to face a sea of faces beaming over their porridge.

depilation

Several days before you leave is also the time to embark on hair removal. Although it may be darkest November, hearty breakers love stripping off and hurling themselves into lakes, lochs and rivers, so be prepared with smooth hair-free skin (and take a spare pair of knickers and T-shirt in your rucksack too). Depilation is one of the most boring areas of beauty, but not without variety in pain and financial cost. If you can bear the pain, waxing is the best and most affordable method for removing hair for a reasonable period of time. Because a beautician can see hairy areas better than you and is more adept at removing the strips, waxing is most effectively done in a salon. If you do not have the time or money for a professional waxing, do it yourself. However, prepared wax strips are not as effective and often do not come off the skin properly if your body is hot. Other methods are listed below, with my probably unwelcome view of how unworthwhile they are.

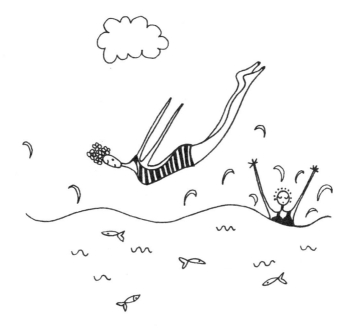

Laser hair removal/electrolysis Prohibitively expensive for most people, this method can be as painful as waxing and has dubious results. Several costly sessions are usually required.

Shaving Although the most convenient, instant solution, bad bristles will develop within 48 hours on the average person. Also, this method is exceedingly uncomfortable for the bikini area.

Depilatory cream Better than ever before in the sense that it is easier to use with the advent of spray formulas, but the cream still smells strange. The effects are not much better than shaving, with regrowth almost identical, if a little slower, and still bristly. However, if you have a low pain threshold or simply cannot stand the thought of waxing, this is a better method than shaving. Another advantage is that the formulas are usually enriched with skin-smoothing ingredients.

hiding your beauty kit

Do not blow your cover: keep your beauty secrets safe and hidden away. Decant small quantites of make-up, cleansers and other supplies into mini pots, Perspex containers or even airtight old plastic containers. If you want to be really furtive, a painting kit can be filled with lipstick and eyeshadow, along with foundation and concealer, and has the added benefit of giving you an air of arty sensitivity. None of these essential items need to be large or heavy. If your sponge bag is microscopic, you will kid your companions into thinking that you are just a down-to-earth natural girl who does not need beauty lotions and cosmetics.

essential beauty kit

- ❤ A small mirror or compact: a self-lighting one will be invaluable for discreetly applying cosmetics and moisturizer in dark tents.
- ❤ A tiny stick of concealer.

- A tiny pot of moisturizing foundation.
- Combined lip and eye block formulated for skiing. The block will make you look like you are taking the weekend seriously, but can be used as a lip gloss and to slick eyebrows in place, as well as to protect against the elements.
- Shampoo and hair conditioner, because you cannot rely on other hearty breakers using it.
- Plasters and antiseptic cream for any blisters or grazes.
- Nail file and tweezers.
- A good sunscreen that offers SPF15 and the four-star maximum UVA protection (see also pages 22–5). Even on cloudy and overcast days you can get burnt, especially if you are sailing.
- Aspirin for headaches, sunburn pain, the sudden arrival of cold or flu symptoms and heart-attack prevention for when you are told that absailing is a part of the weekend's activities.
- A rich dermatological moisturizer for the face and body to keep the drying effects of the sun, wind and cold air at bay.
- Bottle of bath oil or foam or an aromatherapy oil for sneaking a relaxing luxury bath.
- A pack of baby wipes, which will come in handy if running water and washing opportunities are limited or non-existent. Alternatively, invest in a liquid soap that does not require water to wash with.

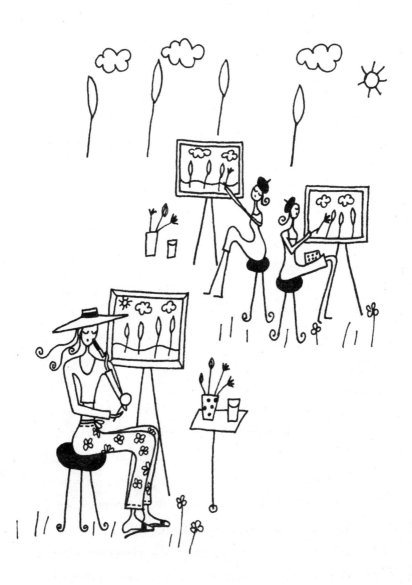

elemental beauty

Battling against the elements should be taken seriously. If you are spending a large part of the weekend walking outdoors, you could suffer from windburn, sunburn and general skin dehydration, even if the weather is overcast and cool. If you are sailing, these problems will be compounded by the salt in the air and the reflection of the sun from the sea.

Whatever time of year it is, protect your skin from UVA and UVB damage by using a high-factor sunscreen see pages 22–5). You only have to look at yachtswomen or mountain-climbers to see that their skin has taken a beating. Take special care to cover your ears, hairline and neck – areas that are often forgotten. Wearing a thick barrier cream helps keep the wind and, to a lesser extent, the cold air at bay. The cream acts like a buffer against dehydration, not simply by keeping the elements out, but also by keeping moisture in.

The skin around the eyes is paper-thin and the first area to show wrinkles and lines. Use a combined lip and eye block to keep it well moisturized. Use the block as an emergency moisturizer during the day – if it is windy, apply it around the eyes to protect against sore, dehydrated and crepey eyes. If the eye area does become very dehydrated, do not overload it with a heavy cream, which could cause puffiness and make the problem worse. A better solution is frequent applications of a light, unperfumed moisturizer, patted on using your ring finger, working from the inside of the eye outwards. To prevent squinting and burning, wear sunglasses.

the sporty make-up look

Creating the appearance of natural sporty health is easier than it sounds. I take smug satisfaction in people asking me why, as a beauty editor, I never wear make-up, though I am usually coated in cosmetics.

Choose a moisturizing foundation if your skin is normal to dry and an oil-free formula if skin is greasy. Oil-free does not necessarily mean that there are no moisturizing ingredients or even oils, but is simply an industry term for products that do not contain certain oils. These formulas give a much more matte finish. Many new formulas offer some sun protection, even up to SPF15, but treat these claims with caution. You are unlikely to wear the foundation thickly or evenly enough to truly protect your skin.

For a concealer, choose one that matches your skin exactly; if in any doubt, choose a lighter shade. The formula should be moisturizing, rather than astringent, and waterproof to protect against exposing spots and veins in rain, snow or hot weather. Despite its slightly heavy texture, a scar concealer will not shift for hours and should be waterproof.

Apply foundation and concealer to well-moisturized skin, only where it is needed (see pages 176–7). Concealer can be worn alone if you do not like foundation or if you have broken capillaries or other blemishes. Do not, under any circumstances, even flirt with the idea of wearing bronzer or blusher, because in the cruel, crisp light of day you will be outed and feel ridiculous. In my experience, walking uphill for more than 15 minutes is enough to turn anyone vermilion, so the last thing you need is extra colour.

Wear a very neutral long-lasting lip pencil or lipstick, applied very subtly and blotted with tissue paper. The pigment will bond to lips for hours. You can keep the colour looking fresh by slicking a clear eye/lip sunblock on top throughout the day, which will add extra sheen and protect the lips from the elements into the bargain. The block can also be used to fix eyebrows in place and give them an extra depth of colour.

If your eyelashes are not dyed, wear a light coat of waterproof mascara on the upper lashes only. For natural-looking defined lashes, apply the mascara by first stroking the wand from root to tip on the top side of the upper lashes. Follow this by applying one more coat of mascara on the upper lashes, sweeping from below.

If you are addicted to wearing perfume, go for a neutral, fresh scent rather than a heavy, seductive aroma. The last thing you will want to do is entice a hearty into your tent with the promise of patchouli and sandalwood.

fake a healthy glow

♥

Hearty types are usually slightly tanned or red in the face all the year round. To help you look the part or to veil a pasty complexion, apply fake tan the night before your weekend begins (see page 31). The newest fake tan formulas give incredibly subtle results. Alternatively, use a sunscreen throughout the weekend that includes a fake tan in the formula.

hearty break hair

Be careful not to choose a hairstyle that mirrors your idea of a hearty breaker – a sporty headband will just look ridiculous if you are clearly unsporty and impractical. The best policy for long hair is to tie it off the face using unfussy accessories. You could strike an earthy pose by using twigs to secure a chignon or ponytail – however, only employ this technique if you are with slightly hippie hearties who will be sympathetic to your 'nature goddess' sensibilities.

If hair looks greasy and you are unable to shampoo it, spray in dry shampoo, holding the container about 12–25 cm (5–10 inches) away from your head (any closer and it will look like lumps of talcum powder). Massage it into the scalp, then brush it out a few seconds later. Alternatively, scatter cornflower lightly and very sparingly into the hair, massage with the fingers, then brush out. Hair will look cleaner and fuller. A little witch hazel can also be dabbed on with cotton wool to help absorb excess grease.

Much seems to be made at the moment of silicone's hair-wrecking qualities, but it does leave frizzy hair smooth, shiny and tangle-free. A tiny bottle of serum will keep hair from knotting and prevents water loss. Apply it to the ends of the hair the morning before venturing out into the elements, or else at night after a shampoo.

the smell of success

The body odour level can become staggering on hearty breaks. If you want to minimize smells, here is a brief rundown of the options.

- ❤ Antiperspirant: Usually with a built-in deodorant, this stops sweating and kills off the bacteria that grow in sweat and create smells.
- ❤ Deodorant: Although deodorant will not prevent you from sweating (which is a healthy response by your body after all), it should keep unpleasant smells away.
- ❤ Deodorant crystal: A must for the new-age addict, this works by suppressing bacterial activity. To apply, wipe firmly across the skin several times.

❤ Bicarbonate of soda: Pat a little under your arms to deodorize and put some in your shoes to reduce odour.

beauty remedies from the kitchen

Hearty types may be fairly puritanical with their dietary requirements, but you should find plenty of instant and highly regarded beauty aides among the shopping. Either volunteer to go food shopping and make sure all the ingredients you need are on the list or rifle through the food supplies and help yourself.

Avocado Packed with nutritious oils, avocado is good for treating dry skin. For a moisturizing facial mask, mash up a ripe avocado, layer it on the face thickly and leave it for 10 minutes, then rinse away. For a hair pack, mash up a ripe avocado with a little olive oil (omit the oil if hair tends to be greasy or fine). Massage the mixture into the hair and leave it for 20 minutes before rinsing thoroughly.

Banana Bananas are wonderfully moisturizing and can be mashed up with a little runny honey and used as a rehydrating face pack to combat the drying effects of freezing wind. Spread the pack over your face, massaging it in well; leave it for 10 minutes and then rinse thoroughly. The mixture can also be used as a conditioner for dry hair; leave it for 20 minutes before rinsing.

Cider vinegar   Dropping two to three tablespoons of cider vinegar into a bath is said to fight fatigue. Apple cider vinegar can also be diluted with water and drunk to boost the immune system.

Cucumber   A mashed-up cucumber applied to the face as a mask will soothe skin and deflate puffiness. A slice of cold cucumber placed over each eye will refresh tired eyes.

Egg   Egg white has a tightening effect and makes a great tired-face reviver for normal to oily skins. Beat one egg white, mix with a little lemon juice, and layer on the face for 10 minutes before rinsing. For a hair pack, mix a whole raw egg and a little olive oil. Smooth over the hair and leave for 20 minutes before rinsing thoroughly.

Honey   Runny honey makes a good facial cleanser and moisturizer, and helps remove dead skin cells. Massage some into the skin with your fingers. Add some warm water and continue massaging. Rinse away thoroughly. For a slightly more exfoliating treatment, mix the honey with some salt or sugar and massage very gently.

Lemon juice   Best for resilient oily skins, lemon juice makes a natural toner. Dilute fresh lemon juice with a little water and wipe it across your face. Lemon juice squeezed into the bath makes an invigorating pick-me-up.

Oats A well-known skin softener, oats are especially good for soothing dry, sensitive skin. For a pampering bath, wrap up some porridge oats in a cloth, hang it from the tap and let the hot water run through the oats. Oats can also be used as a body scrub.

Strawberries Crush some strawberries and mix them with yoghurt to make a skin-smoothing face pack. Strawberries are astringent, so are not suitable for use on sensitive or dry skin.

Yoghurt Yoghurt makes a natural face smoother because the lactic acid in it helps loosen dead skin cells. Simply use plain yoghurt straight from the pot as a face mask.

conquering fear

Absailing, rock climbing and all sorts of rope- and vertical-slope-related activities are frightening. If you suffer from vertigo, then you will not even accept a rock-climbing weekend. If you just need bit of courage to make a bungee jump or walk across a narrow bridge over a fast-flowing river, consider a flower therapy. Although it sounds a bit more Glastonbury than Gore-Tex, flower essences are increasingly popular and you will find countless tiny little bottles in chemists throughout the UK (see also page 136).

The traditional way to take flower essence is to place a few drops on the tongue as often as you like, but drops can also be added to clean spring water and drunk. Rock rose is the one best known for conquering fear.

Aromatherapy oils can be inhaled or added to a bath to help counteract any crazed or neurotic emotions. Some well-recognized calming oils are camomile, frankincense, neroli, lavender, rose, vetiver and sandalwood. Choose the oil you like the smell of most.

Reflexology, shiatsu and pressure-point massage in general are becoming so popular that they are included in some of the most glamorous salon treatments (see directory, page 253). Although reflexology is done on the feet, there are other pressure points in the body which can also help ease overexertion, tension, fear of heights or speed and other ailments.

anti-anxiety-attack massage

1. Find the pressure point on the lower inner wrist by gently feeling between the two bones around the pulse area until you locate an especially tender region.

2. Firmly squeeze your fingers together on either side of the wrist while breathing out.

3. Repeat on the other wrist.

anti-stress massage

1. Press the centre of your palm where it feels slightly tender, breathing out as you press.

2. Repeat on the other palm.

how to be unfazed

- ❤ Don't refuse to do anything that the others appear to be doing easily – you will probably surprise yourself with your bravery.
- ❤ If you are out of breath, draw attention to rainbows, rock formations and interesting flora and fauna. A 'spod type' will be delighted to explain geological fault lines and limestone pavements ad nauseam while you catch your breath and apply some lip salve.
- ❤ Make friends with the 'frightened rabbit' of the group and help them survive the weekend too. You will soon forget your own fears or irritations.
- ❤ Take plasters with you for blisters. Be warned: hearties have an extraordinary disdain for anyone wearing brand-new footwear.
- ❤ If you cannot face another day of frenzied activity, offer to cook supper. Keep the food plain, nourishing and unfussy – the last thing you want is to attract a hopeful hearty imagining endless culinary masterpieces.

how to walk uphill and still look beautiful

A friend of mine who had trekked for days in Pakistani hills was given this tip by her guide. The guide was obviously fed up with taking endless puce-faced, puffing, grumpy tourists trekking who had no idea how to walk.

Take very short, small steps but at a quick speed. The gradient is dramatically reduced and far less effort is needed to climb the slope. Your breathing is kept constant and you will remain calm and cool.

midge attacks

One of the annoying drawbacks about some of the most beautiful parts of the UK is the midge. Midges are mini mosquitoes and live in large communities on moorland and anywhere wild and boggy. They are an even greater nuisance than mosquitoes because they are minute and swarm in great big clouds.

If you are outdoors in a potentially midge-infested area, you must take insect repellent and wear it at all times on any exposed flesh. Mosquitoes do not like lavender, so a little lavender essential oil is a good alternative, but needs to be diluted with base oil before applying it to skin. If you are bitten, take an antihistamine tablet to calm the itching or use eucalyptus cream to reduce irritation.

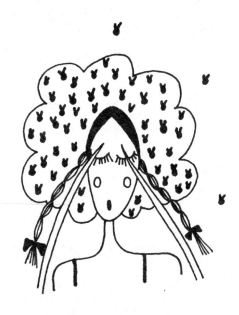

looking on the bright side

Even if you decide an action-packed weekend of sweat, freezing cold streams and long walks is a 'once in a lifetime' experience, look upon it as a fabulous detoxing, cellulite-melting, dermis-cleansing opportunity. The fresh air and activity will do wonders for your skin. City living, stimulant consumption, polluted air inhalation and stress do nothing but damage skin's long-term health. You only have to compare the pallor of a townie with someone who lives in the countryside to know this.

If you are coerced into hearty swims in freezing cold water, think how it benefits your circulation. Plunging in and out of cold water is excellent for getting blood pumping around your body – if only to help it heat up – and this, in turn, helps jump-start sluggish systems. Splashing your face with cold spring water will shrink pores and bring a rosy hue to most skin.

health tips

💜 Because you will be perspiring more than usual, make sure you drink enough water. Even on an ordinary day you should drink at least eight glasses of water, and if you are exercising you should drink even more. Water will hydrate you, enabling muscles to work better, and flush out any toxins.

💜 Avoid sunburn by wearing a good sunscreen and a hat.

💜 Don't drink too much coffee or eat too much bran or other high-fibre foods – you do not want to deal with bionic bowels on a long day's walk.

💜 Wear walking boots if you are hiking or walking long distances. Your ankles will be better supported and there will be less chance of twisting them.

💜 Wet, moss-covered rocks are potentially slippery and dangerous, so take them slowly.

💜 Don't wander off mysteriously on your own. You are not Emily Brontë and leaving your group is irresponsible.

💜 Snakes and other wildlife are very unlikely to bite you. Remember that they are more frightened of you than you are of them.

the end of the day

This is where all the furtive beauty-product packing and preparation pays off. After a day of activity, take the opportunity to sneak in a quick beauty routine (see below). If you are bedding down for the night somewhere reasonably comfortable, a bath or shower should be possible, even if it is a third-hand dip in someone else's water in a bath with enamel so worn away that it exfoliates your buttocks as you bathe.

If you are sailing or camping and there is no opportunity for a shower, use baby wipes to clean your body. They will give you the impression of freshness even if true cleanliness is a million miles away. Combined with the fact that hearties love campfires, candles and other fantastically flattering light, you will be more radiant and alluring than Hiawatha's bride.

evening beauty routine

1. Apply dermatological cream in a thick layer as a face mask and also use it to moisturize the rest of your body.

2. Because your skin is likely to have taken a bashing in the elements, put on more moisturizer than usual to keep water levels up in the skin and help prevent it from being dehydrated the next day.

3. Push your cuticles back with a towel while your hands are still warm from a bath, then rub your nails gently to give them a slight shine.

4. Use dry shampoo if needed (see page 150). Clip hair off the face, or twist long hair into a rustic chignon or low ponytail commune-hippie style.

5. As your face will have had a full day of fresh air, you probably will not need or want to wear foundation. If you do, dab on tiny amounts of concealer and blend in well with your fingers.

6. Define your eyebrows for a bit of sneaky glamour. Do not fill in the entire eyebrow, but just add a little eyebrow pencil at the outer edges where the brows arch over the brow bone.

7. Dab on some lip gloss.

8. Use a shimmer stick to maximize the effect of camp firelight catching your face. Similar to a huge lipstick, they are available in either silver or bronze shades. Apply only a tiny dab where you want your face to catch the light, then blend in. The hearty party will be so mesmerized that they will overlook a few charmingly human eye bags and spots the following day. ...

chapter six

the weekend city break

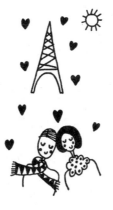

Two friends returned from a mini-break in Venice. 'How was it?' I asked brightly. 'Did you feel like Helena Bonham Carter in a velvet-swathed Merchant-Ivory film?' 'Not exactly,' said the boyfriend slowly. 'I was bitten by the sort of mosquitoes that I would have thought could only evolve after a nuclear disaster. My bites were so bad, I could barely walk.' 'He was pathetic,'

snapped his girlfriend. 'I know he hates walking around galleries, but it was ridiculous. We seemed to spend most of our time discussing antiseptic cream with Italian pharmacists.'

The problem with weekend city breaking is that you are under tremendous brochure-lifestyle pressure. It is almost impossible to imagine a weekend in a major European city without thinking of advertisements targeted at retirement couples in leisure clothes or carefree, madly-in-love couples in clinches under famous landmarks. Apart from the fantasy, the reality is trying to pack everything you want to do into a limited period of time. Overexcitement and tiredness from travelling and sightseeing conspire to destroy any veneer of serene and sophisticated beauty – whether it is strange bodily rashes or smudged, greasy make-up.

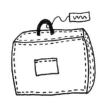

prepare ahead

Stockpile medical remedies to halt potential disasters, such as colds, diarrhoea or blisters from walking. Trying to explain the finer symptoms of a blister or mucus problem to a non-English speaker is not only deadly dull for them but does not necessarily guarantee the right remedy. For attractiveness purposes, take pills or powder – squirting nasal spray on a Bâteau-Mouche is one of the least glamorous ways to spend a day in Paris. The combination of different water and hotel soap may trigger skin complaints. If you are prone to rashes, eczema or other stress-related skin problems, take the usual creams and pills you ordinarily use.

Before you embark on your break, invest some time in giving yourself a few pampering beauty treats. Take an evening to body scrub, wax your legs and underarms, and paint your nails. If it is spring or summer, make a fake tan the icing on the cake (see page 31). In warm climates, you will be able to walk around bare-armed and -legged, and a well-applied fake tan will help you feel healthier and more relaxed about revealing an otherwise pale, dull, wintry skin. If you cannot face applying it yourself, call a spa or beauty salon and book yourself in for a fake tan treatment. The treatment should also include a body scrub and possibly a massage, which will add to the lovely luxury of the planning stage.

skin protection

In sampling the delights of a big city, you will also be indulging in polluted air. Ultraviolet rays, which cause 80 per cent of skin ageing, combine with pollution to make a particularly potent skin and health wrecker. Wearing a moisturizer that offers SPF15 as well as an antioxidant in the formula will help protect against the ageing effects of sunlight and pollution, though not sunburn. There is a wide choice of protective 'city blocking' lotions and creams available that shield the skin from pollution. Some are not formulated to moisturize the skin so you may have to add a moisturizer on top.

Even in chilly climates, skin is at risk from elements such as wind, and changes in temperature and cold air speed up water loss. Sightseeing all day can be a dermal challenge, particularly if you have dry or sensitive skin. Help keep water levels in the skin high by applying generous helpings of moisturizer, and a moisturizing foundation if you need it. Keeping the water trapped in the skin with a thick layer of moisturizer reduces the chances of chapped or cracked skin and even the most simple formula will be effective.

If you are somewhere hot, you must wear a sunblock instead of an SPF moisturizer. Sheer yet high-factor sunscreens are available, which can be worn under make-up as an extra protective layer and do not make the skin look as greasy as ordinary sunblocks. If you have oily skin, consider using a microsponge oil-absorbing foundation or moisturizer. Fairly recently, cosmetics companies started including microscopic sponges in their grease-controlling products. These mini sponges absorb sebum from the skin and keep it looking fresher for longer. The microsponges are found in everything from serum that you apply like a grease blocker under make-up to tinted moisturizer, foundation and even powder. Some of the oil-absorbing serums can be dabbed on top of make-up to take away shine.

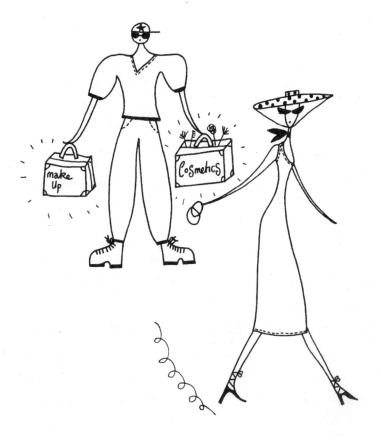

city break make-up kit

Unless you have a strong manservant or you are happy to haul a heavy bag of cosmetics and beauty lotions around with you, pare your beauty needs down to the barest minimum. This does not mean you have to look anything but ravishing, but there is no need to take unnecessary bottles and jars. Try to choose products that will do several jobs at once.

two-in-ones

One of the cleverest inventions in recent years is the two-in-one powder foundation. Prototypes were once fairly simple – a creamy foundation that gave reasonably heavy coverage and a powdery-looking finish. But now there is the most fabulous choice of textures, colours, finishes, skincare benefits (from moisturizing to grease-absorbing) and even cooling formulas for the summer.

Some of the most natural-looking products are very light and gel-like, which are preferable to the traditional opaque versions. Most come with a mini sponge that is used to swipe the foundation over the face. Match the foundation to the jaw line rather than to any other part of your face: an exact match will appear to melt and fade away on the jaw. Skin tends to be either pinky-blue or yellow in tone and you should try several tones to see which one works best.

Another doubling-up product is a combined eye and lip pencil. Great big thick crayons and 'multisticks' are available in assorted hues that can be used as eyeliner, eyeshadow, lip colour and blusher. These crayons or sticks tend to be soft and creamy, making them extremely easy to smudge for a subtle effect. A good alternative to a 'multistick' approach is to use a neutral rose-brown lipstick in a similar way.

long-lasting cosmetics

To retain the appearance of beautiful skin for hours and hours, choose the right long-lasting make-up. Long-lasting foundations were originally quite dry and dull in texture and finish. Unless skin was smooth in the first place, areas that crease regularly, such as around the eyes and mouth, looked slightly lined after a few hours. The opaque finish was also quite unnatural. I remember wearing what I thought was a rather fabulous new foundation to a party and was asked if I had had flu. Enter the new generation of latest long-lasting formulas, which offer more 'glow' than the pioneer formulas, give sun protection, keep moisture levels up in the skin and can last for 12 hours or more. They also contain clever little ingredients, such as microbubbles that roll across the skin as the foundation is applied so the formula feels silky-smooth. Long-lasting lipsticks have also improved tremendously. Originally rather dull and drying, they now look and feel smoother and last just as long. Some even contain pigments suspended in a special base that preserves the shade (lipstick colours can alter slightly after they have been on the skin for some time).

---

base note

If you are terrified that foundation will be noticeable when you are outside in the cruel daylight, invest in a formula that offers 'photochromatic pigment' technology. The photochromatic pigments adjust to different light colours and intensities, creating an undetectable foundation.

---

beauty kit checklist

- Insect-repellent spray, plasters and antiseptic cream.
- Diarrhoea pills and cold remedies.
- A hair dryer and travel plug: most standard hotel hair dryers take far too long to dry hair.
- Bubble bath or oil: having a glamorous, aromatic bath is fundamental to the luxury factor, and the versions offered by hotels are far too small and usually lacking in top-quality bubbles and aromas.
- Scented body cream or lotion, preferably one in your favourite scent.

- ❤ Papier poudre for greasy skin: probably one of the oldest and most useful cosmetic inventions, papier poudre are finely powdered leaves of paper that are excellent at absorbing excess oil and leaving the skin looking lightly powdered.
- ❤ Eye gel: hot hotel rooms and travelling may create huge eye bags.
- ❤ Toner or a mixture of rose-water and witch hazel to keep skin looking and feeling fresh.
- ❤ 'City block' pollution shield or moisturizer with SPF15 or greater.
- ❤ Leg spray or gel.
- ❤ Combined mascara and make-up remover.
- ❤ Compact two-in-one foundation or a long-lasting version.
- ❤ Lip and eye pencil or multistick.
- ❤ Mascara.
- ❤ Blusher and/or bronzer.

refresher course

If you are boarding a plane or train straight from work, or are planning on going out as soon as you arrive, you will not have time for a bath, shower or generally tittivating time. Follow these steps to freshen up quickly and, although your skin will not be as spotlessly clean as you would like, you will feel less dishevelled and look less tired, leaving you feeling and looking better for longer.

1. Thoroughly cleanse and tone your face, then reapply your make-up.

2. Keep your make-up simple. Use a compact foundation or concealer to even out the skin and then add a little colour with a light bronzer or blusher.

3. For limp hair, apply a little hair spray to the roots of the hair and massage your scalp vigorously with your fingertips to thicken out the hair and add volume. Then brush it into your normal style.

4. For static hair, spray some hair spray onto a comb and pull it slowly through the hair.

5. For greasy hair, use a dry shampoo (see page 150). Take care to cover your shoulders, or brush away any spray that falls out of the hair, because dry shampoo can look suspiciously like dandruff.

6. Drink as much mineral water as you can while travelling. You will feel more clear-headed when you go out for dinner the first night and the next morning when you will want to be as sprightly as possible.

7. When you arrive, put some toner and eye gel in the mini bar for refreshing skin and combating puffy eyes.

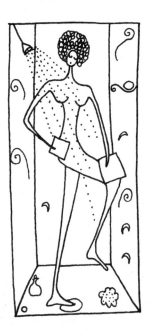

the first morning

Travelling and general cavorting the night before has probably ensured you have woken up feeling less than lovely. If you are feeling tired, a morning bath will just send you to sleep, so have a shower instead. To wake you up, use a flannel soaked in cold water as a body mitt. Using long strokes, sweep the flannel from the feet up towards the heart and from the hands in towards the shoulders. This is the direction your body's waste-disposal system, the lymphatic drainage system, works and the mitt will help jump-start it into working more effectively.

Black rings under the eyes are likely to be made worse by dehydration. At breakfast, drink plenty of water rather than multiple helpings of coffee, which will only dehydrate the body further. If the bags under your eyes are enough to rival a leather-luggage shop, soak two cotton wool pads in chilled toner and place them over the eyes for about five minutes. Your eyes will feel instantly refreshed and because toner helps close pores, the puffiness will also be reduced. Eye gels, like toners, contain astringent ingredients to help produce a cooling and anti-inflammatory effect. Do not use gel or toner if the skin around the eyes is sore, as they may irritate it. Instead soak two pieces of cotton wool in cold water, squeeze out the excess and press gently over the eyes. Leave for five minutes, then remove and smooth on a little moisturizer.

hotel bathroom warning

Hotel beauty kits must have been invented by a mad person. Unless you are 5 years old or a pygmy, the mini nail files are far too small to use properly. The shampoos never seem to work as well as the most ordinary high-street formulas and the shower hats can only be relationship-destroyers. However hilarious you and your loved one are, trying on a bath hat will do nothing for your allure. If you need to pin your hair up in the bath a tousled ponytail or French pleat is much better.

coping with style xenophobes

Do not try to emulate European style. European women are brilliant at looking classic and cool because they have been trained from birth by their mothers and you cannot compete with them. Instead, turn heads by swanking around in your favourite piece of clothing, leaving a trail of unusual fragrance in your wake.

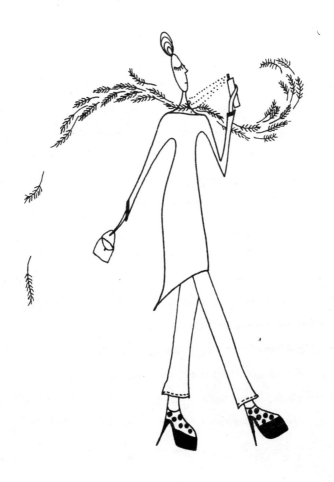

If we Brits tend to lack the meticulous approach to beauty that many European women have, it is only to our advantage. An English friend of mine told me, after she had been living in Paris for four years, 'Even if I tried to get ready as slowly as I possibly could, by the time I'm fully dressed, made up and coiffed, a French girl would just about be putting on her tights.'

I am not suggesting that all of us do not take trouble with our appearance, but one withering 'up-down the body' eye flick from a tight-lipped Parisian woman can leave even the most relaxed among us wanting to shrink into the nearest *poubelle*. Content yourself with the knowledge that English eccentricity and originality cannot be matched anywhere else in the world, and the same goes for beauty. Stick to being a fresh, natural, lovely creature and leave the permatanned, logo-emblazoned, anorexic Eurosnoots to battle it out among themselves.

how to not look like a tourist

- ❤ DON'T wear sporty clothing and baseball hats, or clothes emblazoned with logos.
- ❤ DON'T wear shorts: if you want to visit churches, you will not be let in some of them.
- ❤ DO take a tiny camera. Disposable ones are remarkably good and more discreet than a paparazzi-style camera that can get stuck in other tourists' armpits in crowds.

- ❤ DO keep your hair brushed and off the face (using sunglasses as a headband, if necessary) – tourists typically have sweaty hair plastered to their scalps.
- ❤ DON'T complain. Wherever you go in the world, the biggest complainers are the British.
- ❤ DON'T eat ice cream in the street.
- ❤ DO carry your guide book in your bag and only refer to it when necessary. However beautiful you may look, a guide book is an invitation to be ripped off by taxi drivers, boatmen and others providing a service.

becoming the 'not so natural' english rose

Unless you are a supermodel, remaining flawless-skinned and gorgeously groomed after a day of sightseeing and shopping is about as likely as middle England giving up double glazing their houses. To fake English Rose skin, you must get your foundation to look as flawless as possible. Many of the latest innovations contribute to a far more natural, and far less detectable, look (see pages 56–9). Apply foundation with your fingers in very small quantities. If you use a cosmetic sponge, 'wipe' in the same direction as the fine hair on your face grows. Areas that need a little more cover should be built up in layers. Do not be tempted to give yourself a healthy glow with foundation: use bronzer or blusher for this. The most important tip is to blend the foundation almost obsessively into the skin. Professional make-up artists create flawless skin on models by dabbing, blending and using a rocking action with their fingers to press the foundation firmly onto the skin. Areas that give the game away are around the nostrils, outer corners of the eyes and under the eyes, so use a little cotton wool bud to smooth away any excess foundation here. For any areas that need heavier cover, apply concealer on top of the foundation (concealer applied first will be wiped away when the foundation is applied). Take a little time to get the foundation right, but it should not take more than five minutes.

Powder can look a bit too heavy, especially in daylight, so avoid it. Add a little blusher or bronzer to your cheeks or where the sun would naturally hit the face to create a look of glowing health. Choose a bronzer or blusher that has a more natural matte, browny-pinky tone, rather than an orangey-gold tone. Avoid cosmetics with sparkly particles because they will be too visible and artificial-looking in daylight.

Groomed eyebrows give a face a polished appearance without looking a bit contrived. For a sleek, defined brow line, put some hair spray on a finger or brow brush and slick eyebrows into shape. Clear mascara is also good at holding brows in place. If you want to define your eyebrows, use a pencil that is a shade lighter than your brows and only apply colour to the outer V that forms over the brow bone. This will give your face a fresher, more open look. Use a neutral, matte eyeshadow all over your eyelids, right up to the brows. Choose a shadow that is a tiny bit lighter than the skin above your eyes. The shadow will give eyes a fresh, bright quality and will be undetectable. A beige eyeshadow or exact match for your skin colour will not create the same 'freshening' effect. Finish with light coats of a waterproof mascara that will resist smudging from the wind, watering eyes and perspiration. To achieve undetectably coloured lips, use a long-lasting lip pencil shaded all over the lips, then slick a lip salve on top to prevent lips looking dry.

undercover experiments
for shrinking violets

In a foreign location you can be a little more exotic than you might be back home. If you feel like wearing more dramatic eye make-up or a darker lipstick than usual, this is the opportunity to experiment. You will feel more anonymous, and if you like the effect, you will have broken it in. There is nothing more conversationally deadening than the remark 'Oh you look nice; you look slightly different'. The resulting self-admonishment of 'Oh no, is my lipstick really that obvious? Does it look tarty?' can be avoided on a city break where you can indulge in some beauty practice and get over any new shade phobias.

feet first

Feet deserve special attention on city breaks. Walking and standing all day, particularly in hot weather, makes feet and ankles swell. Leg sprays and gels have a fantastically cooling yet fairly superficial effect. If your feet are killing you and ankles that were once finely chiselled delicacies have become stout piano legs, without so much as a flicker of an anklebone, put your feet up. Lie on the bed with pillows under your feet or lie on the floor with feet flat against the wall, your legs higher than your head, and use a leg gel or spray. After 10–20 minutes, your feet will be ready for an evening of dancing.

fresh-smelling feet

- ❤ DON'T wear synthetic shoes.
- ❤ DO put odour-eating foot shields in shoes.
- ❤ DO spray your feet with deodorant or antiperspirant or dust them with talc before putting on shoes; or rub a cut lemon over them – although I find this rather sticky.
- ❤ DO shake some talcum powder inside shoes.
- ❤ DON'T cover your feet in scented body lotion after a shower if the weather is hot: feet will just feel hotter and sweatier in shoes.
- ❤ DO remove your shoes at the same time as someone else; that way you can blame the smell on them.

resisting taste sabotage

Every city and their inhabitants have certain weaknesses. In Spain, for example, it is gold handbags; in France, it is disgraceful hair accessories – some of the hair bands are so enormous they could almost be installed as soft furnishings. Before long, seemingly by osmosis, you find yourself buying and wearing the sort of things maiden aunts gave you for Christmas in your teens. Another potential disaster spot is perfume. Increased heat and aspirations of being drenched in mystery can prompt us all into buying the most unlikely and unsuitable scents – especially if you smell something that seems to fulfil these fantasies trailing down a street.

city guide

❤ **Edinburgh, Glasgow and Dublin**

Because the light is either cold, clear and bright or dull and grey, it is likely to be cruel and will illuminate imperfections. Stick to long-lasting matte textures and natural colours, avoiding any shimmery or yellow-toned make-up. Style warning: avoid national costume of any kind, such as kilts or tam-o'-shanters, or bargain Scottish or Irish woollen knits in cable patterns or bobbly tweedy wool. Do not buy Celtic brooches or jewellery unless you know what the symbols mean.

❤ London

An anti-pollution sunscreen is a necessity here, particularly in summer. Cultivate a healthy glow to counteract all the pasty, grey, cross faces you will see around you (see page 62). Style warning: do not buy Union Jack hats, T-shirts, socks or other wares emblazoned with nationalistic symbols. To avoid robbery, do not wear expensive jewellery or watches and do not wear rucksacks on buses or tubes. Avoid gothic-looking make-up, unless you are going to Kensington Market and are at least 40 years old.

❤ Amsterdam and Stockholm

The light is variable, so use a foundation that offers photochromatic technology (see page 245). Make-up should be natural, but you may like to introduce a little more eyeliner or a slightly funkier lipstick to give you a slightly mysterious edge over the Scandinavians. Style warning: avoid over-groovy accessories and buying huge clumpy shoes to increase your height so you can look the natives in the eye.

❤ Paris, Madrid, Rome

The temperature may be higher here than at home, so use a light SPF tinted moisturizer, or an oil-free one if you have greasy skin, particularly if the weather is hot and sunny. Employ 'fake' natural English Rose make-up techniques (see pages 176–8) all day and night because restaurants can be brightly lit in the evening. Style warning: avoid Euro-style middle-aged elegance. Sunglasses with huge logos and too much bronzer will not convince the locals you are indigenous.

♥ Vienna

The light here is similar to England, but can be stronger in the summer. Make sure you wear an SPF tinted moisturizer. Style warning: do not waste your Euros on checked felt clothes or anything beige.

♥ Prague and Budapest

These cities tend to be dull and grey, especially in winter. Keep your complexion looking rosy with cream blusher on the apples of the cheeks and use a moisturizing make-up if the weather is cold. Style warning: avoid appliquéd clothes, tarty shoes with trousers, chain-store jewellery and mid-1980s make-up.

crise de foie

This useful French expression describes an overload of rich food. Having a rather spartan heritage, gorging on cream-drenched food, rich seafood and cheese can be a bit of a shock for the Brit body. The best way to give your liver a rest without bypassing any culinary delights is to increase your intake of still water. Keeping everything nicely diluted will help you feel better quite quickly.

If you have *crise de foie*, it also pays dividends to drink like Europeans rather than Anglo-Saxons (less quantity and more quality drink), rather than pouring as much alcohol down your throat as you can manage before the bars close.

flagging energy antidotes

The combination of travelling, overheated hotel rooms and rushing around all day drains the body's reserves. Boosting energy levels with sugar, caffeine and other quick-fixers is a short-term solution, but bad for your breath and hopeless for long-term health and beauty. Most minerals and vitamins should be obtainable from eating a healthy, balanced diet, but you may suffer from deficiencies in certain essentials, such as potassium and vitamin C. Typical potassium deficiency symptoms are lethargy and insomnia. Insufficient vitamin C creates a depressed immune system. Smoking kills off vitamin C in your body every time you have a cigarette, which is why smokers are more susceptible to colds and flu than non-smokers. If you are feeling uncontrollably grumpy, take magnesium, which is believed to help soothe ragged nerves.

Another simple way of improving energy levels is to eat a fruit-and-vegetable breakfast and lunch, and save gourmet guzzling for the evening meal.

chapter seven

disaster days

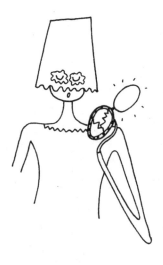

It has happened. Whether you have danced like John Travolta on speed the night before and you now look like one of Dracula's victims or you have tried a temptingly packaged rejuvenating face cream that has failed to live up to its promise, a gasket has blown in the beauty department and you are looking less than lovely.

I have had my share of beauty disasters. Being referred to by my friends as 'potato face' for the duration of a skiing holiday is high up the list. Thanks to the combination of a wrongly prescribed steroid cream and the sun-drenched ski slopes, my face swelled to such proportions that I had to wear a balaclava for days. I have also had cold sores so large that it looked as if I had inserted a pebble into my upper lip – and these examples are just the start of it. A similarly afflicted friend and I call each other 'dermo twins' – we both suffer from sensitive skin and between us we have most skin nightmares taped.

On the whole, though, beauty disasters are generally far worse and more obvious to the stricken individual than to anyone else – in fact, the whole culture of 'bad hair days' was probably invented by a devilishly successful shampoo salesman. But rather like ghosts and other spooks, beauty disasters are horrifyingly real if you believe in them.

mad woman frizzy hair

Because frizziness is caused by excess water, humidity is often the culprit. The best antidote is to increase the moisture level in the hair using a rich conditioner or serum. This prevents water in the atmosphere sneaking into the hair shaft and causing curling. There are also good anti-frizz or hair-relaxing products on the market. In a real emergency, massage a tiny amount of hand cream into your hands, then stroke through your hair to keep mad tendrils looking smooth and polished.

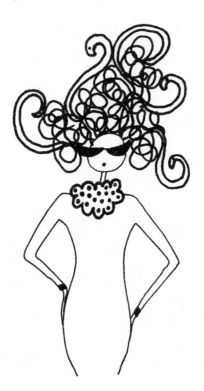

seriously static hair

Static hair is often caused by using a dirty hair brush. If your hair is still flyaway after giving your brush a good clean, spray a comb with hair spray and gently comb it through your hair.

fine, floppy, hippie hair

Unless you are spectacularly beautiful or a 1970s revivalist, limp hair pasted to the head is very unflattering. As someone who has spent her life (or at least part of it) teasing limp, fine hair into a thicker mop, the following techniques seem to work. Apply a hair-thickening spray generously (at least 10 squirts) and comb it through your hair. Always dry your hair upside down. For real body – a sort of modern-day backcomb without the 1960s flavour – take small sections of hair (no more than half a little finger in thickness) and twist each one gently about four times, then split it down the middle, pulling the bunch apart down to the root.

As a quick-fix solution for limp, greasy hair, a dry shampoo is unbeatable. The trick is to hold the can at least 30 cm (12 inches) from your head for a fine spray and a less 'chalky' finish. Massage your scalp to help the shampoo absorb the grease, then brush it out with a dense-bristled brush.

ingenious bad hair tip

♥

If your hair looks dreadful and you can't do anything with it, wear sunglasses like a headband. If you feel a bit of a prat – especially if it is deepest-dark winter – get some cheap fake spectacles and use them the same way; this will also give you an air of intelligence and slight mystery.

split ends

The obsession with split ends is one of the most boring phenomenons since the invention of craft fairs. However, if you are in paroxysms of horror about having them and do not have time to get your hair trimmed, use an extremely heavy-duty hair conditioner that claims to repair split ends. Although it will not mend them forever, the hair shafts will be coated with a thin layer – most likely of silicone – to give the impression of healthy hair. Tiny quantities of hair wax or serum (or even a pea-sized amount of hand cream) applied to the ends of the hair will also help, giving the illusion of hair bursting with moisture. Although we are all encouraged to believe we can become mini salon stars, your hair will look and feel a lot better if you do not overdry it – wait until your hair has almost fully dried naturally before using a dryer.

perm disaster

No sympathy here I am afraid. Unless you are going for a bit part in a television soap series, what on earth are you doing perming your hair? As it grows out you will only look like a poodle that has been around the block a few times. If, however, you have been seduced by a perm and disaster has struck, it is not a catastrophe. Ask a reputable hairdresser to see if they can restyle it, but otherwise accessorize as you have never done before. Console yourself with the thought that you will be providing entertainment for your friends for a few weeks and that you will never do such a foolhardy thing again.

cold sores

There is no getting away from the fact that cold sores are horrible, painful and noticeable. There is very little you can do to cover one up. If the sore has not broken over your lip line, follow the make-up artist's adage that you should never emphasize both the eyes and the lips. Concentrate on making up your eyes and leave your lips nude – perhaps just apply a small slick of lip gloss to counteract any dryness – and you will be amazed at how the cold sore seems to fade away.

If the cold sore has broken over the lip line, use a concealer to paint the inflamed skin to match the rest of the skin. Applying powder directly to the sore will only exaggerate it and, if the sore is dry, make it look even drier. For immediate treatment, use a cold sore medication slavishly. For long-term protection, take lysine supplements each day. Lysine is an amino acid which counters the chemicals found in certain foods (such as peanuts) that encourage cold sores.

flaky lips

Anyone who has suffered from seriously flaking lips knows that almost all the beauty tips do not really work. Rubbing lips with an old toothbrush or flannel makes lips flake even more and become sore into the bargain. Do not use a moisturizer unless you are desperate, because in my experience they just make sore lips worse. Many lip salves seem to make dehydrated lips drier and before you know it, you are addicted to reapplying them. Because the really greasy formulas seem to be more drying than most, the best solution is to apply plenty of non-greasy lip salve every 30 minutes, if need be. The protective top layer of skin on the lips will soon become stronger and you will be able to give up lip salve altogether after about three days, with just the occasional slick when you really need it. Tea tree oil lip salves are especially good and also seem to prevent cold sores developing. Avoid wearing long-lasting and matte lipsticks, which can be very drying;

instead, choose a moisturizing lip gloss in a light colour, which will help give a smoother, glossier impression.

horror movie eyes

If you are prone to dark rings, get sufficient sleep and step up your water intake, but avoid caffeine. In Chinese medicine, dark circles are regarded as a sign that the body is not clearing itself of impurities effectively. In the long-term, drinking at least a litre of mineral water each day will help flush out toxins, but covering the dark circles is the most immediate remedy.

If your skin is golden in tone, use a yellow concealer under the eyes. If your skin is bluey-pink in tone, choose a slightly pink shade. Some of the latest concealers are

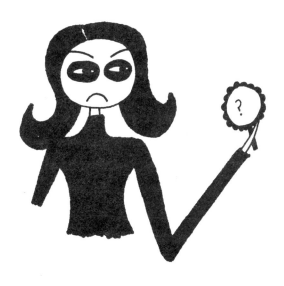

undetectable and, thanks to volatile silicones in the formulas, give a silky slip rather than the heavy pasty finish of older versions.

Use a very light-textured concealer under the eyes, because after a few hours of laughing or scowling the make-up will settle into fine lines around the eyes, making you look older and more tired. Avoid powdering directly around the eye socket for the same reason. Subtly blended dots of concealer or a pale highlighter at the inner and outer corners of the eyes will give tired eyes a new lease of life. A pale pink or lilac matte eyeshadow brushed just under the eyes will also help counter dark circles and perk the eyes up.

fag-ash Lil face

Whether you are a smoking enthusiast or just stayed up too late, your skin will start to look ashen if it is deprived of an opportunity to recover. 'Beauty sleep' was not given its name for nothing. Research shows that skin repairs at its fastest rate and gobbles up nutrients most intensively during the night. To speed up skin repair and restore a nice healthy bloom, use a moisturizing night cream (see pages 108–11). Creams that contain antioxidants or vitamins help improve skin repair; oxygen creams help increase radiance (and are especially good for smokers, who starve their skin of oxygen); and exfoliating creams help to rejuvenate dull and pasty complexions. The new enzyme-based facial exfoliants, most commonly containing papaya enzymes, are not only very gentle on the skin but really effective. A face pack, whether it is a home-made version or a commercial preparation, will also help jump-start your skin into life.

quick beauty fix for fag-ash Lil face

Try this refreshing exercise to get blood circulating around a pale, pasty face.

1. Stand with your legs 50–100 cm (2–3 feet) apart, or wider, and stay stable.

2. Keeping your legs straight and hands on your hips, bend from the waist, out and down towards the floor.

3. Put your palms flat on the floor and keep gently stretching downwards.

4. Slowly creep your hands forward to give yourself a bigger stretch. Breathe deeply for 5–10 breaths, depending on how comfortable you feel.

5. Move your hands back towards your feet, then put them back on your hips and slowly stand up.

make-up face lift

❤

If you look exhausted, don't apply make-up – eyeliner, eyeshadow or mascara – on the lower eyes because it will just drag your face down. Dab a little pale ivory highlighter under the brows and on the inner corners of the eyelids, smudging outwards. Finish by applying a little mascara and eyeliner to the top lashes only.

summer evening beauty

Picture the scene: romantic candles are being lit, Italian-style salads have been carefully drizzled with olive oil, the sun is still out and it is a perfect summer's evening – until you put on make-up. There seems something rather drag-queenish about wearing evening make-up in the summer; strong golden light has a mischievous habit of rendering even quite subtle make-up dazzlingly obvious. The key is to avoid any product with shimmer or sparkle or any kind of heavy make-up because the chances are you will be a little tanned (whether natural or fake) and making the skin tone look even is more important.

Thanks to all the glamorous associations of lipstick, you should be able to get away with wearing any shade or texture. A simple but chic application of lipstick gives the impression that all you need to do to look glamorous is wear lipstick, and no-one will know you have spent an embarrassing amount of time perfecting your skin.

summer make-up tips

❤ Opt for a sheer, moisturizing foundation if skin is dry to normal, or an oil-free formula if skin is greasy.

❤ Mix a little tinted moisturizer (make sure it is matte, not shimmery) with the foundation for a sheer effect.

❤ Applying thin layers of foundation on top of thoroughly scrubbed, moisturized skin will make it look more natural and even.

❤ Take special care to avoid too much foundation or concealer around the eyes.

❤ Unless you are obsessive about using powder, do not apply it on top of foundation. Most of the new foundations and tinted moisturizers look more natural when they are worn on their own and do not need 'setting' with powder.

❤ For a radiant glow, brush a highlighter over your cheekbones, brow and chin – and shoulders and collarbone if you are showing them off. Choose a creamy highlighter with a mother-of-pearl texture rather than a shimmery white one. An eyeshadow will do exactly the same job and should be cheaper.

❤ To add more colour to the face, rub a little cream

blusher onto the apples of the cheeks and blend well; however, be aware that blusher will look awful and fake if you have a tan.

♥ Keep eye make-up simple by applying a matte cream or neutral-coloured eyeshadow over the lids and blending it with a fingertip up to the brows. The colour should be more concentrated at the centre of the eyelids and fade away up to the brows.

♥ Brush your eyebrows into shape and seal with clear mascara; alternatively, squirt some hair spray onto an old toothbrush and brush it through the brows.

♥ Use a tiny amount of eyeshadow to add colour to your eyebrows – choose a colour that is slightly lighter than the natural shade of your brows so they do not look too heavy.

♥ For natural long-lasting lip colour, use a lip liner all over the lips and add a slick of gloss on top to prevent your lips looking dry.

english rose skin

Rather like rosebuds, English Rose skin can be relied upon to look fresh and lovely for an unfair length of time. However, it is prone to oversensitivity, dryness and even eczema. To prevent potential disaster days, keep the skin's moisture levels up. This means avoiding alcohol-based toners, astringent cleansers and light moisturizers. If your skin is particularly dry, apply twice your usual amount of moisturizer like a face pack and let your skin soak it up. Always keep a good protective layer between your skin and the elements by wearing slightly more moisturizer than you think you need.

sallow, olive skin

In many ways olive skin is a gift from Mother Nature. It may look sallow, or even a little green, when you are tired but it is generally resilient – a huge advantage over English Rose skin, which reveals late nights quicker than a pea creates a bruise under a princess's mattress. Olive skin tends to be normal to oily, and although it is usually less sensitive, it is prone to open pores and an unhealthy pallor. The best complexion perker is a fake tan (see pages 29–31) – use one and you will switch from green to golden delicious in less than an hour.

Olive skin can also be perked up with a yellow-based foundation or golden-toned pre-foundation primer. This skin type tends to be most sallow around the eyes, so do not use a pink or pinky-beige foundation or concealer – it can make the skin look grey. A tinted moisturizer blended in meticulously will also give the illusion of freshness. Dust with bronzer, rather than blusher, and avoid green or blue eyeshadow or 'cool' blue-toned lipsticks, using warm pinks, browns and corals instead.

bruises and scars on the body

If you want to reveal bare flesh but have noticeable scars, bruises or broken veins on your legs, do not try to conceal them with ordinary make-up. The pigment in ordinary concealers is not dense enough to provide even coverage on these areas and will leave the scars or bruises looking grey and the rest of the skin looking unnatural.

You can buy specially formulated waterproof scar concealer from department stores and specialist make-up shops. Because the texture of these concealers tends to be matte and heavy, apply them by patting the colour on. Allowing the product to warm slightly on the skin first makes blending easier.

burst veins and capillaries on the face

Cover visible veins and capillaries with a microscopic amount of birthmark or scar concealer or, if they are not too pronounced, an ordinary moisturizing concealer. Using an index finger to rock the concealer into the skin will help it stay in place longer.

Do not be tempted to use blue or green 'cooling' foundations – they are quite difficult to use and rarely look natural. If you cannot find an exact colour match, choose a concealer that is one shade lighter than your skin tone, then dust the area with powder.

rash solutions

Rashes can be caused by hundreds of different things, from stress to allergy. A rash is the body's defence system kicking in to ward off some sort of enemy. When the immune system goes on 'red alert', histamine is produced by the body to fight the aggressor. Unfortunately, if we overreact, whether through allergy or stress, unnecessary histamine is produced. Taking antihistamine tablets should reduce, if not eradicate, rashes in a few hours, but if you need emergency cosmetic cover, different techniques are called for. Red rashes can be dulled by applying green or blue concealer, or even foundation. Apply the colour, little by little, in very thin layers and dust with powder for a matte finish. If the rash is a reaction to a cosmetic or feels itchy, avoid irritating the skin further by applying foundation or concealer. Instead, dab on a low-dosage hydrocortisone cream and follow with a light dusting of powder.

As a general rule, if you have dry skin or rashes around the eyes, do not try to cover them up – the rash will become more obvious when covered by even the lightest layer of the most high-tech concealer. If the rash is very dark, but not raised or dry, invest in a birthmark or scar concealer. The high pigment content of these rather cement-like formulas give total – and, in some cases, waterproof – coverage. As with any concealer, apply with a brush or little by little using a fingertip.

eczema

Eczema is an overreaction of the immune system, which is why sufferers often get hay fever and asthma too. Once skin starts to behave abnormally, it loses the plot about its real role in keeping irritants out. The skin sends more antibodies to the problem area, an eczema patch or rash, and this increases the redness, flaking and even weeping. The 'barrier' function of the skin needs to be kept working as well as possible. Mild eczema can be dealt with fairly easily by keeping moisture levels high to allow skin to recover and regain its natural equilibrium.

In my view, and experience, loading the skin with steroid cream over a period of time (even just days) is an effective temporary solution but it does not get to the root of the problem and can actually make skin more vulnerable to allergy and overreaction. If you have bad and frequent attacks of eczema, consider trying Chinese medicine. Although this form of treatment can take months to work, the results are impressive. Over time, a Chinese doctor should be able to 'rebalance' your system so that everything works more efficiently, rather like tuning a car engine. You may also find that Chinese medicine increases your body's overall energy levels. The treatment usually involves drinking Chinese tea, which tastes revolting, or taking numerous tiny pills, which are much more convenient and pleasant (see directory, page 253).

aid for eczema

- ❤ Don't ever use an astringent, alcohol-based cleanser or toner – even if your skin feels greasy.
- ❤ Frequently apply a rich, unperfumed dermatological cream with spotlessly clean fingers.
- ❤ Never put hydrocortisone (steroid) cream on your face unless you have first consulted your doctor and been instructed to do so.

aeroplane face

Ever wondered why film stars wear shades when they are disembarking from a plane? Because they look dreadful. A very particular beauty disaster happens after a long flight: you emerge looking tired and crumpled and, however much you use your complimentary toothbrush, you have killer breath. Although leaving a plane looking ravishing is unlikely, you can minimize the damage by keeping your body properly hydrated and your skin clean and well moisturized.

Trying to wash your face in one of those little aluminium sinks is one of life's more irritating experiences. By the time you have collected enough water in your hands, the tap has stopped flowing. If you try to fill the basin with water, you will probably find someone else's toothpaste swirling around in it. A good alternative method is to use a water spray to wet your face and then wipe it several times with a good toner. Follow this with double the amount of moisturizer you would ordinarily use and your face will feel clean, refreshed and soft.

inflight tips

- ❤ Avoid wearing make-up on the flight.
- ❤ Apply a moisturizing face mask in a clear, see-through formula that can be worn without anyone noticing.
- ❤ Take a water spray and a small bottle of toner with you to cleanse your face.
- ❤ Use an eye cream-gel: it feels refreshing and should also help moisturize effectively.
- ❤ Drink plenty of still mineral water.
- ❤ Avoid fizzy drinks, unless you want to become a spare turbo jet.
- ❤ Avoid alcohol – it will dehydrate you.
- ❤ Provided your skin is not sensitive, baby wipes are good for refreshing skin and for a surreptitious wipe of the armpits in the aeroplane loo.
- ❤ Take some breath fresheners with you or a mini bottle of mouthwash to help combat flight breath.
- ❤ Although you cannot prevent your feet from swelling during the flight, ease the pain by wearing a soft, comfortable pair of shoes and by taking them off as soon as you get on the plane.

grease-ball face

Coping with oiliness is easier in winter; in summer perspiration increases sebum production and attracts dirt. Use an oil-free moisturizer as well as an oil-absorbing foundation to counter excess oil. Long-lasting foundations are particularly well suited to oily skin, so consider investing in one of these if you need extra cover. You can also use oil-absorbing face powder or papier poudre (see page 170) to dab on when needed.

If your skin is very greasy, try some of the latest skincare products that reduce oil production. Tests have shown that over time they can help reduce the amount of oil produced by the skin. Using face masks or scrubs that claim to absorb oil will not only hoover up excess grease but will also give your skin a fresh feeling, thanks to stimulating ingredients like menthol in the formulas.

serious spots

If you are suffering from bad spots, see your doctor. Skin is considered to be suffering from acne if you have as few as four spots at any one time. If your doctor is not helpful, do not be dissuaded – ask to be referred to a dermatologist. Alternatively, contact the Acne Support Group (see directory, page 253). Use cleansers and moisturizers formulated for oily skin and an oil-free spot concealer to cover them.

doughy, untoned body

If your pasty body is soon to be exposed by encroaching summer months or a beach holiday, either invest in kaftans or try the following beauty routine.

1. Exfoliate your body with a moisturizing body scrub (see also page 28). Although you can use a mixture of sea salt and light olive oil, ready-made formulas generally give better results.

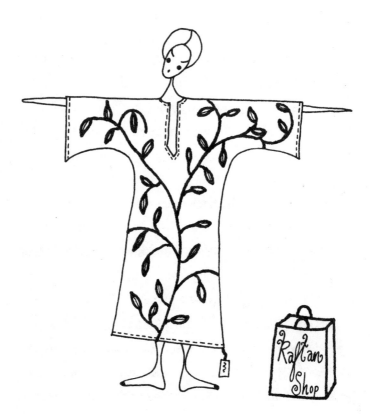

2. Rub skin vigorously with a warm damp flannel. This will remove any residual scrub and give the skin an amazingly smooth finish.

3. When the skin is still slightly damp, apply generous amounts of body lotion, massaging it in thoroughly.

4. Next apply fake tan (see page 31). A golden tinge is better than a dramatic change of colour. If you are worried about streaky colour, choose a tinted formula so you can see where you have put it.

5. Paint your toenails a dramatic, vibrant colour to detract from the rest of your body.

lovely face, bad breath

Eat fresh parsley. Chlorophyll is a key ingredient in many breath refreshers and is found in abundant qualities in parsley. Avoid smoking, eating spicy food and drinking red wine, all of which are well-known contributors to halitosis.

smelly feet

Few people have fantastically smelly feet, but there are plenty who have easily avoidable problems. Wearing the same pair of shoes without letting them dry out is an easy way to build up odour. Ideally you should allow two days and nights between shoe-wearing sessions. Spraying feet with deodorant will help suppress odour-generating bacteria. Dusting feet with talcum powder, or bicarbonate of soda if you are really stuck, will also help combat smells.

broken nails

If your nail splits, simply trim all your nails to the same length and concentrate on growing strong nails by frequently applying a nail-strengthening cream. To mend the split quickly, take a tiny thread of cotton from a strand of cotton wool (so small that you can hardly twist it) and put it in the split. Pull away the excess cotton, then paint your nail with clear nail polish or a base coat.

nail fungus

This is the beauty problem that dare not speak its name. If the top part of your nail starts to come away from the nail bed, you have nail fungus. The best treatment is drops of neat tea tree oil between the finger and the nail bed twice daily. The affliction can persist for months but you must continue using the tea tree oil long after the nail has recovered. Nail fungus is rather like a lingering ex-boyfriend: there is no predicting its persistence or when it will rear its enthusiastic head again.

chapter eight

future happiness

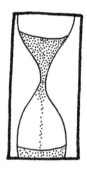

'It's all the biggest load of crap I have ever come across,' screeched a lawyer one evening over dinner. 'All creams are exactly the same and you just pay for the packaging and advertising.' 'And do you know,' trilled another instant cosmetics expert, 'all the cheap brands are made in exactly the same factory as the expensive ones? It's the biggest rip-off of all time!' They rolled their eyes towards me as if I had been breeding hamsters for vivisection or stealing money out of wallets from women with crow's-feet.

The anti-ageing market throws up some fantastic cynicism as well as utterly unrealistic expectations. The mother of a friend of mine told me how thrilled she was by the prospect of some minor plastic surgery (while I was eating Parma ham): 'To be honest,' she whispered in a confidential tone, 'I'm going to be 60 [mouthed] next year and I'm not prepared to look it – I don't want to be, I don't feel ready. It's as simple as that.' The fact that she believed that she would look radically different, several thousand pounds later with slightly more pouty lips and less droopy cheeks, was beyond me, but her view is an increasingly common one.

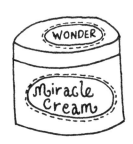

what does it really mean?

Each year, the anti-ageing skincare market swells. Beauty journalists can just about get their heads round the trends in technology, the ideas that appear to be original and the not-so-good ones that are trumped up beyond their merit, but anyone else with a vaguely interesting life does not have the time or patience to trawl around department-store cosmetics counters and chemists' shelves looking for exactly the right cream for their needs.

One solution is to declare that the whole thing is a clever marketing con and you are better off sticking to something cheap and simple. Some dermatologists would certainly agree with this. 'All anyone ever needed was petroleum jelly,' bellowed one specialist down the phone when I interviewed him. He is right, of course, if you look at skin from a certain angle. There is nothing medically wrong with skin that is slightly rough, oily or heavily wrinkled. It functions; it looks as it should; it performs its intended role of protecting the rest of the body from damage, whether from ultraviolet light or bacteria – yet it may not look its best.

The appearance of ageing skin is a subjective topic that is made more complicated by clever marketing and different ideas on what constitutes good skin. Do you want plump, firm skin? Radiant skin? Smooth skin? Wrinkle-free skin? Or to fade uneven pigmentation? The questions are endless. The most foolproof way to assess a cream is to look at the ingredients and see how they tally with the claim it makes. Of course, most creams contain combinations of different ingredients targeting different problems, but there are general 'camps' they fall into: antioxidant creams to fight sun and pollution damage; exfoliators for smoother, fresher-looking skin; or collagen supporters to help skin retain its firmness.

can you really see the difference?

In order to make claims that an anti-ageing cream works, cosmetics companies put their products through stringent tests. Results can seem impressive. In fact, the results of the 1998 SUVIMAX survey (a long study of the effects of antioxidants applied to the skin) proved that antioxidants not only protect the skin against ageing but also help reverse damage, albeit in very small amounts. However, the only way you will really find out whether a certain cream improves your particular skin is to try it. Most brands will give you samples to try, so do not be shy about asking for some. Although you should not expect miracles, if you do not see any improvement, the cream is obviously the wrong one for you so do not waste any more money on it. Creams only work for as long as you use them, so after a few days of giving them up, their positive effects will cease.

free radicals

Free radicals are the main cause of photoageing (sun damage). They attack lipids, the fats in the skin that keep skin moisturized and soft, destroy collagen and elastin and contribute to wrinkles, dryness and skin cancer. Free radical skin damage is rather like an unhealthy love affair. Free radical molecules are made naturally in the body during the cell oxidation process. In normal, healthy circumstances they find electrons, like men or women find mates, to make them feel complete. Free radicals only become dangerous when they cannot find a free electron to bond with and they smash up a healthy skin cell in order to get their electron – like a lover might damage a marriage or an existing relationship in order to find a partner. Despite the fact that the original free radical cell has been immobilized in finding a mate, the damaged body cell now creates more dangerous molecules.

Antioxidants, such as vitamins A, C and E, are rather like benevolent dating agencies, which provide electrons for these otherwise destructive molecules and calm them down. Antioxidants are the equivalent of the police, patrolling the skin cells and rendering any rogue oxidized cells powerless. Although some vitamins are well-known antioxidants, the two terms are not interchangeable. Other antioxidants often included in anti-ageing creams are green tea and grapeseed extract.

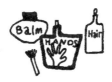

vitamin-based creams

The idea that you are feeding your skin with vitamins is very appealing, but if vitamins taken orally are good for general health, why not for skin too? When vitamins are ingested, the body grabs the 'goodies' first, whereas if they are applied directly to the skin, the theory goes, improvements should be more noticeable.

Vitamins are organic molecules required by the body for growth and function and they also help protect and repair damage in the skin, nails and hair. In most cosmetic preparations their 'anti-ageing' role is touted primarily as a protector against free radical damage to healthy skin cells, however, certain vitamins do have more specific roles. Vitamins A, C and E are three of the most widely used antioxidants in skin creams and each performs a slightly different function.

vitamin A

Vitamin A is considered to be the normalizing vitamin and comes from the reinoid chemical family, which includes retinol, retinal, retinoic acid and carotenoids. Our skin needs vitamin A for healthy skin development. The vitamin helps maintain the skin's firmness by guarding against collagen breakdown. It improves collagen production, helps the skin retain moisture and increases the skin's thickness (skin thins with age).

However, vitamin A is rather like Frankenstein's monster. It may have great positive qualities but it does more harm to the skin than good if it is used wrongly. Overuse can result in rashes and sensitivity to light. Originally, the most powerful vitamin A skin treatments were prescription-only creams. Acne patients prescribed Retin-A were noticed to have reduced fine lines and wrinkles, and although Retin-A was never officially marketed as an anti-ageing cream, dermatologists did prescribe it to treat ageing. Another vitamin-A-derived acne treatment, Renova, was eventually given FDA approval and sold as an anti-ageing cream. Both creams are strong, and should only be used under dermatological supervision.

Retinol is another powerful vitamin A derivative which, fairly recently, has become 'flavour of the month' in anti-ageing skincare. It is the key ingredient in a number of anti-ageing creams sold over the counter. According to cosmetics companies, retinol creams can help reduce fine lines and improve firmness as well as lighten age spots and even out skin pigmentation. However, just like the more powerful vitamin A predecessors, retinol cream or serum should be applied at night and a sunscreen must be worn during the day. Some cosmetics companies claim retinyl palmitate has a smoothing, brightening effect on the skin and the ingredient is included in 'radiance enhancing' creams and in a variety of different cosmetics. However, it does not carry the same sunscreen warning and has a less dramatic effect (if any, according to some opinions) on the skin.

vitamin C

Because vitamin C is not made in the body, we depend on eating food that contains it to help provide fuel. Although vitamin C has been found to have a positive effect on the health of skin, it is likely to be used up by the body before it reaches the skin. Applying it directly to the skin helps improve collagen production and protects the skin against damaging ultraviolet light. Because the vitamin is unstable, becoming ineffective once it comes in contact with water, fresh, active vitamin C tends to be sold in phials of powder and serum, which then need to be mixed together and used immediately. Alternatively, the vitamin is encased within high-tech microbubbles, which dissolve once in the skin, releasing their cargo.

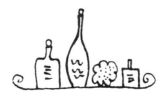

vitamins E, F and K

Vitamin E is a good preservative and has been used for years in face creams to prevent them from oxidizing. It is no surprise, then, that the antioxidant effect was seized on by cosmetics companies and the vitamin is widely used as a skin preserver and antioxidant. Think of vitamin E as the hippie of the antioxidant gang: it is a skin smoother and soother; it keeps moisture in the skin; it helps heal wounds and is anti-inflammatory. Vitamin F is a good moisturizing agent, which helps the skin remain strong and effective at retaining moisture. A more recent addition to the list of skin improvers is vitamin K, which is included in many creams to improve circulation in the skin and it is found in some eye creams. However, this vitamin's qualities and its possible side effects appear less known and, for this reason, some cosmetics companies have not yet included it in their skincare formulas.

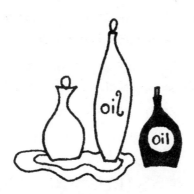

key anti-ageing vitamins

Vitamin A derivatives, such as retinol, are anti-ageing and anti-wrinkle treatments. They are used to treat the serious effects of ageing and are suitable for mature skin. Vitamin A may cause sensitivity in the skin when it comes in contact with ultraviolet light, so don't embark on the use of a vitamin A product unless you are prepared to wear sunscreen every day.

Vitamin C is a skin saver and firmer; it protects against ultraviolet damage, encourages the production of collagen and may also improve radiance.

Vitamin E is a good basic skin preserver that should be used in copious quantities all through your life.

how to spot vitamins in a skincare formula

You will not necessarily find vitamin E or vitamin C in the ingredients lists in creams, even if they claim to be antioxidant vitamin creams. Annoyingly, slightly more scientific terms are used, and here are a few to help you decipher the blurb.

- Vitamin A – retinol, retinal, retinoic acid, carotenoids.
- Vitamin B – niacin, pyridoxine, riboflavin, pantothenate, thiamine, biotin, folic acid, cobalamine.
- Vitamin C – ascorbic acid, ascorbyl palmitate.
- Vitamin E – tocopherol and derivatives; for example, tocopheryl acetate.
- Vitamin F – linoleic acid, arachidonic acid, linolenic acid.

acid-based creams

Acids wear away at the surface of the skin, melting the 'cement' between skin cells and speeding up the skin-shedding process, making the skin appear fresher, smoother and younger-looking. They were hailed as a great skin revolution in the early to mid-1990s. The best and most finely tuned formulas were successful and are still selling well, however, the 'me-too' products that were carelessly constructed and too aggressive for many skins to tolerate fell from grace when other anti-ageing ideas hit the market.

Varieties of acids used in the formulas are AHAs and BHAs (see pages 240 and 241–2), both from plants; glycolic acid, from sugar; and lactic acid, from milk. The term 'fruit acid' is interchangeable with AHA and was probably used because it sounded more palatable to a consumer market increasingly obsessed with natural ingredients. BHAs possess larger molecules than other acids, which make them, theoretically, less irritating because they cannot sink as deeply into the skin. Salicylic acid is the best-known and most successful BHA in the market place. Using lactic acid to smooth the skin is not a new invention – Cleopatra was famous for bathing in milk to keep her skin smooth for her lovers and the benefits of using yoghurt as a face mask are widely regarded.

enzyme formulas

Enzymes act as exfoliants to smooth and brighten the skin and are often found in gentle facial exfoliants as an alternative to harsh grains. Papaya and pineapple are two popular enzymes. You may also find that some skin-firming creams contain enzyme activators and these boost the skin's collagen-rebuilding system.

plumping out the skin

Although this sounds rather like your face is like an old mattress, bear the analogy in mind. Collagen and elastin fibres are the 'springs and stuffing' of skin and as we age the fibres break down. Although the process is inevitable, it is speeded up by sun damage from UVA rays, and for this reason never believe that UVA-only sunbeds are worth going on – they may be less likely to burn you, but you will turn into a prune in no time. Smoking is another collagen and elastin destroyer. Not only is cigarette smoke charged with free radicals (see page 212), but smoking also destroys vitamin C supplies in the body and vitamin C is an important collagen-repair ingredient.

Years ago 'collagen' creams were simply luxurious moisturizers, but now collagen- and elastin-building formulas are rather more impressive. Many of the latest versions contain ingredients that actually speed up or improve the skin's natural collagen and elastin systems. Oxygen moisturizers also help smooth and improve the appearance of the skin, and these are particularly good for smokers who starve their skin of oxygen every time they light up (see also page 110). Although some specialists claim that too much oxygen can contribute to premature ageing, unless you are a triathlon champion the chance of incurring this sort of damage is unlikely. In my experience, oxygen creams do make a difference and give the skin a lovely healthy bloom.

a little extra help

Serums, oils and face masks are the icing on the cake of anti-ageing skincare, helping to boost an otherwise simple daily skincare routine.

Serums are fluids that are packed with skin-improving ingredients. Just as daily skincare is unbelievably diverse in everything it offers, so too is the choice of serums, whether you want to improve collagen firmness, remove dulling dead skin cells or fight free radicals. Serums should be applied under ordinary moisturizer. Because most are quite strong, they only need to be used two or three times a week or at times of the year when your skin needs all the nourishment it can get, such as in winter when you will be fighting off colds and a duller-looking complexion. Always read the manufacturer's instructions carefully.

Specially pre-blended and diluted essential oils are another way of giving your skin some extra help. Because essential oils contain molecules that are small enough to enter the bloodstream, they can improve skin circulation at a deep level. Face masks have come a long way since the days of mud packs and other cement-like formulas and are now simply another way of giving your skin a moisturizing, firming, tightening boost. More fun to use than ordinary moisturizer and generally cheaper than serums, they also help fight the war against dehydration and other enemies of youthful-looking skin.

all-natural self-help

Sleep is one of the most important anti-ageing steps you can take. Skin repair is at its height at night when the skin is not busy defending itself against sunlight, pollution and other environmental invasions. Give your skin plenty of rebuilding and recovery time and get a good eight hours of

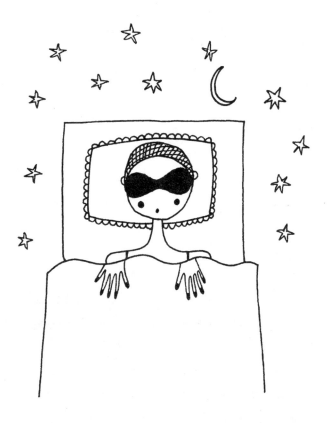

sleep a night as often as you can. The best skin repair time is apparently between 11 p.m. and 3 a.m.

As well as sleep and exercise, protecting your skin cells with a balanced diet is an obvious way to keep skin looking healthy. The following foods are all rich in nutrients and are often used extracts in skincare products: avocado, vitamin-C-rich berries such as strawberries and cranberries, blueberries, broccoli, cabbage, carrots, citrus fruits, garlic, grapes, spinach and tomatoes. Drinking green tea may also help boost your body's skin defence system.

blocking ageing rays

Long-term skin damage is caused mainly by UVA rays, and not as much by UVB, the 'burning', rays. UVA penetrates deep into the skin, damaging the support structure of collagen and elastin fibres. Because such a huge proportion of lines and wrinkles are caused by sun damage, wearing a sunscreen all the year round is worth doing. Choose a sunscreen that offers UVA protection as well as UVB cover (see also pages 22–4). If a sunscreen offers UVA protection, this will be represented as a star rating: four stars are the maximum protection against UVA rays and mean that the amount of UVA screen is as high as the SPF number in the formula. To block the ageing rays, you should choose an SPF15 plus a four-star UVA protection. Do not be fooled into thinking that a low SPF combined with a four-star UVA protection will be a great anti-ageing formula – it simply means that the UVA protection is as limited as the UVB. Many new moisturizers now give SPF protection, but little mention is made of screening against UVA, so these moisturizers will not help protect against ageing 100 per cent.

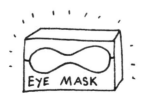

EYE MASK

crinkly eyes

However much the rugged Marlboro man might crinkle up his eyes and stare knowingly into the distance, sadly, a female version does not have the same attractiveness. For women, fine lines and wrinkles are seen as beauty faults, which are to be prevented for as long a time as possible. Women's skin is thinner than men's and ages faster. The skin around the eyes is some of the thinnest of all and has limited oils and less fat, which prevent it from looking fresh and lovely.

Eye creams are basically mini moisturizers, but lighter in texture. They may include extra benefits, such as antioxidants, skin soothers and even light-reflecting pigments to reduce dark shadows. Eye creams, rather than gels, can help slow down the dehydration process. Eye gels are formulated to deflate bags and give a cooling, refreshing sensation but rarely claim to moisturize the skin. You may be able to find an eye cream-gel, which will feel cool when applied and help deflate bags and retain moisture. If crow's-feet have already begun to surface, use a moisturizing eye cream, which will help the wrinkles look less pronounced. Avoid applying powder, heavy concealer or foundation around the eyes, which will just accentuate lines. Do not be tempted to apply AHA or retinol creams close to the eyes unless the packaging specifies them for that use – they will be too strong and could cause a rash.

how to prevent crow's-feet

❤ DON'T smoke: smokers always have worse crow's-feet than non-smokers.
❤ DO drink plenty of water.
❤ DON'T wipe toner over the delicate skin directly under the eyes: it is too dehydrating.
❤ DON'T use eye gel to keep wrinkles at bay.
❤ DO use a moisturizing eye cream that includes light-reflecting pigments.
❤ DO go Jackie O by investing in a large pair of glam sunglasses that provide total protection against ultraviolet light for your eyes and the skin around them.
❤ DON'T sunbathe without wearing a sunscreen specially formulated for the eye area.

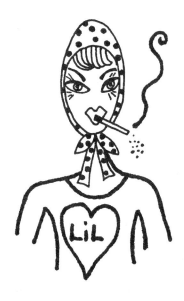

anti-ageing make-up

Some of the latest foundations promise to make you look younger. This is quite a significant claim because some foundations can make you look older, settling unflatteringly into fine lines and wrinkles around the eyes and accentuating uneven areas of skin. This can be made even worse if your skin is dry and the formula is oil-free.

There are two approaches to anti-ageing make-up and sometimes both elements are combined to give you a super luxury treatment. The first approach is including anti-ageing ingredients, such as fruit acids, antioxidants and other skin preserving and protecting ingredients, in the formulas. The second approach is packing the formula with ingredients that give the illusion of younger-looking skin, such as moisturizing ingredients to keep the skin looking fresh and dewy and light-reflecting pigments to help the skin appear luminous. If you decide to use a 'treatment' foundation – a formula that claims to brighten and improve the natural state of your skin, with fruit acids for example – make this your only 'anti-ageing' measure initially. Too often, anti-ageing novices are overenthusiastic in their use of exfoliating cleansers, serums, moisturizers and foundation, which can overload the skin, causing sensitivity and rashes.

Many foundations will offer some protection against the damaging effects of ultraviolet light, particularly if they include titanium dioxide. However, to get any real sunscreening benefit you would need to apply the foundation evenly and thickly. If you want to protect your skin against sun damage and wear foundation at the same time, a better idea is to moisturize your face first with a good-quality sunscreen (many of the latest formulas contain an impressive ingredients list) and then apply a foundation on top.

Some concealers formulated for the under-eye area, occasionally referred to as 'highlighters', can be used to create the illusion of youthful, radiant skin. Apply these concealers in areas that need brightening: around the eyes if they look tired and pink; under the eyes to conceal dark circles; or on the cheekbones and temples to help skin catch the light.

Lipstick formulas can also give the impression they are anti-ageing and in a sense they are – some offer SPF15 protection as well as antioxidants and other skin-improvers. However, as lipstick only too easily wears off, the only way you will really get any benefit from these formulas is to constantly reapply them. Keeping moisture levels up, whether with lipstick or a lip salve, is the recommended course of action. As soon as moisture levels drop, the skin is more likely to dehydrate, crack and develop fine lines.

choosing youth-enhancing make-up

♥ If your skin is dry, use a moisturizing foundation rather than powdery or oil-free formulas.

♥ For a little extra colour, mix a tinted moisturizer with your foundation.

♥ Avoid an exfoliating formula if you are using other anti-ageing creams or serums – you may overload your skin.

♥ Choose formulas that contain light-reflecting pigments or photochromatic technology (see pages 244 and 245).

anti-ageing make-up tips

♥ DO apply foundation in thin layers, little by little, rather than an unnatural thick layer.

♥ DO blend foundation over the eyelids as a primer for eyeshadows and to give a fresh look to the face.

♥ DON'T apply concealer or foundation all over the under-eye area – just dab it lightly on areas that are a little dark or pink.

♥ DON'T ever use bright eyeshadow colours.

♥ DO stick to neutral-coloured eyeshadows in shades of brown and grey.

♥ DON'T wear eyeliner all around the eyes or along the lower lashes; apply it only very subtly to the outer corners of the upper lashes.

♥ DON'T wear dark lipstick colours – lips look thinner and

lose their colour as you get older and dark colours enhance this.

- ❤ DO wear a pale slightly shimmery colour of lipstick to make lips look fuller.
- ❤ DON'T wear a matte-textured lipstick, which can make lips look dry and old.
- ❤ DO use blusher on the apples of the cheeks – pink tones are better than peach as you get older.
- ❤ DON'T brush powder right under the eyes. Even if you think this will help reduce the appearance of bags, lines and dark circles, it will just make your skin look dry and even more lined.

washing away your youth

We have all been drilled into enthusiastically cleansing, toning and moisturizing our faces, but do not imagine that this is guaranteed to keep your skin looking radiant and young. In fact, overwashing with the wrong cleanser can actually do more harm than good. It can weaken the skin's natural defence function and leave it open to attack from heat, wind, cold and pollution, which in turn can lead to increased sensitivity and even allergy.

Deciding which cleanser to buy can be complicated. Not only can you buy cleansers that are packed with any number of glamorous-sounding ingredients that claim to leave the skin more ravishing, but cleansers are also available in so many different forms – ranging from bars and gels to lotions and creams. And that does not even include the accessories you can buy, such as facial brushes, pads, cloths and scrubs. The bottom line is that you have to cleanse skin to remove grime and make-up, but without stripping the skin of natural – and helpful – oils. Traditional soap is perfectly capable of cleaning the skin well, but because it is alkaline and the skin is acidic, it can strip the skin of its thin protective outer layer.

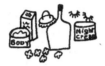

If your skin is dry, choose a creamy wash/wipe-off formula. Gels are usually more drying and better suited to oily skin. Rinsing your skin thoroughly is one of the best things you can do in the whole cleansing process. No matter how swanky or expensive the cleanser, leaving traces of it on the skin will not do your skin any good. Toners are probably the most easily dispensed-with stage of the skincare regime, but are worth using to leave the skin feeling refreshed and clean and to ensure that no grease or cleanser is left on the skin's surface. If you are trying to hold back time, use toners containing glycolic acid or other anti-ageing ingredients, but be careful not to use too many other anti-ageing products. Although you might have to endure an intolerable hard sell from cosmetics staff, discuss your other skin products with them before buying an expensive toner. If you are already using an anti-ageing serum, moisturizer and foundation, you will not achieve any more benefits by using an anti-ageing toner, and you could push your skin over the edge. A good toning tip is to splash your face 20 times with cold water morning and evening after cleansing and before moisturizing. This will help close pores and contributes to a lovely, natural 'bloom'. However, if you have very delicate, dry, English Rose-type skin, which is rarely combined with open pores anyway, do not do this – your rosy complexion could turn into a network of minute broken capillaries.

---

rose-water toner

If you want an inexpensive basic toner, ask your local chemist to make up one of the following recipes.

For normal to dry skin: ⅓ rose-water, ⅓ distilled water and ⅓ witch hazel.

For normal to greasy skin: rose-water and witch hazel in equal quantities.

For sensitive skin: rose-water and distilled water in equal quantities.

---

fighting the onset of flab

As we get older, the metabolism slows down and weight inevitably piles on. Exercise and healthy eating help prevent excessive flabbiness in the skin, but they do not necessarily guarantee it. Most adults in the UK are overweight and in the USA the statistics are even worse, yet eating disorders are on the rise too. The healthiest thing you can do is accept your natural shape and adjust your intake to suit your metabolism. Staying within an acceptable weight and increasing exercise will help you feel younger and more energetic.

Eating well is common sense. If you need plenty of food to keep your energy levels up and your temper under control, do not restrict your diet too much. If, however, you are on the podgy side, do not try to eat everything on your plate at every meal. One of the best diet tips I can offer is to stop eating when you no longer feel hungry. So many of us are undisciplined about following this rule, and once our snouts are in the trough we have to guzzle our way through whatever is before us. If you feel you might offend your hosts, discipline yourself not to worry. In many cultures it is polite to leave a little food on your plate as it shows that you have eaten your fill. Do not ever treat yourself with food. Food should be eaten when you are hungry and for its nutritional value, not for getting through a failed relationship or overstepping your overdraft. You are not a dog and do not deserve crisps or chocolate-covered drops as a reward for anything. Much better treats are lipsticks, hair clips or mini bottles of bubble bath.

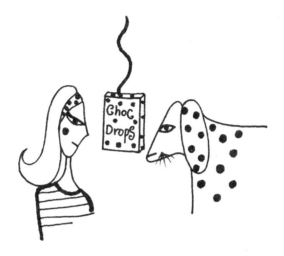

Yoga and pilates are two forms of exercise that elongate muscles and help the body look leaner. You only have to look at yoga teachers for living evidence of yoga's benefits: they look younger and have firmer bodies than people of the same age. In my view, overly muscled aerobic queens are a far cry from the natural shape of women.

Purely cosmetic treatments may have some effect and will probably make you feel, if not look, better. Anti-cellulite creams will not banish existing cellulite but they will smooth and tone the skin and reduce the uneven appearance of cellulite. Salon or spa treatments are even more effective, but remember that you will have to invest in a number of treatments (see also pages 16–18). Like facial creams, body lotions also include antioxidants, AHAs and other exfoliators to leave skin looking smoother and firmer.

the bust zone

I remember sending one friend of mine for a luxury bust treatment who reported that the therapist referred to her bust as 'the area' in rather puritanical tones. French women, by comparison, think nothing of lavishing all sorts of lotions and potions on their chests. The idea that Europeans care for their bodies feet upwards and English with toes curled upwards is still generally true: we tend to concentrate on our faces and forget everything else. Bust creams and gels aim to improve the firmness and softness of the skin but cannot honestly be expected to lift boobs that jangle somewhere around the stomach. A much more effective anti-ageing strategy is to keep the skin on the chest and around the collarbone beautifully cared for. This area is the first to show signs of years of sun damage and should be protected vigilantly with a sunscreen of at least SPF15 on all sunny occasions.

neck firming

A cream that firms the neck is rather optimistic, as we all know what happens to necks in the end. Neck creams are really only for the rich and worryingly obsessive (although I am sure French women would disagree). Polo necks and scarves may eventually be the best solution to ageing necks, but sweeping massage movements up the neck and out along the chin will help defy gravity. To do this, work from the collarbone upwards, using a generous helping of moisturizer.

age spots

Many retinol-based products (see pages 108–9 and 246) claim to fade age and pigmentation spots, and this benefit is offered in anti-ageing face creams as well as in many hand creams. If age spots truly bother you, discuss the matter with a dermatologist who may be able to prescribe a pharmaceutical vitamin A derivative cream, which will have a more dramatic effect than any cosmetic preparations.

seriously sneaky tactics

There are a number of salon and surgical treatments that give your face a younger appearance. Personally, I think they should be approached with caution, not particularly for the health risks (they are widely practised and controlled), but because the psychological effect is more insidious. Thinking you might need a non-surgical face lift may seem a benign way to improve your looks, but it could pave the way towards a dependence on more extreme methods, which may make you look slightly different to who you are. In the end, a good mental-health approach to ageing will serve you better than relying on the effects of any cream, treatment or surgery. If, however, you are interested in these anti-ageing measures, here are a few non-surgical options.

Non-surgical face lift This method is not as radical as it sounds. Muscle tone and circulation in the facial skin are speeded up using microcurrents, which is most commonly done by stroking conductors gently over the skin of the face. Some people swear by the non-surgical face lift but, like most beauty treatments, a number of sessions will give the most impressive results. You will find this treatment offered in most good spas and beauty salons throughout the UK.

Botox injections Frown furrows can be removed by injecting Botox, a plant bacterium. The facial muscle is prevented from moving so the frown line melts away. The result is not permanent, and the effects of the initial injection will wear off after three months. Although a Botox treatment leaves the face looking calmer and possibly younger, it can make you look a little inexpressive. Concern over the long-term effects on facial nerves and muscles is also now coming to light.

Collagen injections   A well-established line-filling treatment, collagen injections can freshen up a tired-looking face for up to six months, although the collagen eventually breaks down. There is a small chance of an allergic reaction.

Hyaloform and Hyalangel injections   Far less likely than collagen to cause allergy, these injections last for a similar length of time. Both Hyaloform and Hyalangel are hyaluronic acid derivatives, which is a natural moisture ingredient produced by the skin.

chapter nine

beauty-speak translation service

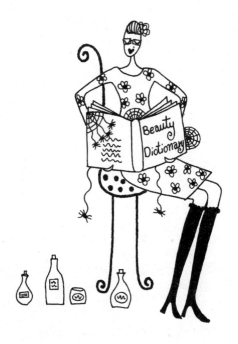

Flick through a glossy magazine or listen to a cosmetic ad on television and the same clever but fairly vague phrases are slipped into the advertising 'speak'. Does 'reduces the appearance of cellulite' mean that existing cellulite will be diminished or does it mean that future cellulite will not be as bad as it otherwise might? If the latter is the case, how can you possibly measure the benefit?

Thanks to the stringent advertising rules, cosmetics companies cannot get away with out-and-out lying about the effects of their products, but there is no doubt that clever wording, however legally correct it may be, does increase expectation levels. Being realistic about what a pot or tube of cream can achieve is the first essential step, but understanding the 'beauty speak' will help sort the chaff from the grain. An added advantage is that it will equip you with all the vocabulary and knowledge you need to hold forth, dropping into conversation technical – often rather meaningless – beauty words to convince any mean-spirited souls that beauty is at least as serious a subject as economic theory, philosophy or car engine sizes.

AHAs, alpha-hydroxy acids, are anti-ageing skin-brightening ingredients. They include lactic, malic, citric and glycolic acids, and although derived from different sources (lactic is from milk and glycolic is from sugar), they all work by loosening dead, complexion-dulling cells from the surface of the skin. This forces the skin to make new, fresh, ultimately better-looking skin cells, resulting in a younger-looking complexion. Although AHAs were all the rage in skincare in the early 1990s, they have been used for years, albeit in cruder forms; for example, a natural yoghurt and honey face mask is a classic moisturizing AHA treatment.

Alcohol-free products should be read as suitable for normal to dry, but particularly dry, skins. Alcohol is astringent and good at removing grease, however it can be too harsh for fragile, dry skin which needs more soothing, moisturizing ingredients. Traditional toners were once solely alcohol-based, but now there are plenty of gentle, moisturizing formulas.

Antioxidants charge around in the skin saving healthy skin cells that would otherwise be 'oxidized' – think of them as skin soldiers. An oxidized cell, rather like a vampire, produces dangerous free radical molecules that sneak around the skin system destroying other nice, kind, healthy cells. Antioxidants are sometimes referred to as 'free radical scavengers' because they neutralize aberrant molecules. The ones most commonly used in skin treatments include vitamins A, C and E, green tea and grapeseed extract.

Aromatherapy is a rather unspecific term when applied to oils or products. Anything can be called aromatherapy if it smells nice and makes you feel good, but the term does not mean the product contains high-grade essential oil (see page 243). Cosmetics companies sell ready-blended aromatherapy products which can be used safely in the bath or on the skin. The percentage of genuine plant extract can be deduced by the ingredients list: if the extract is one of the last few ingredients listed, you know that there is very little of it in the formula.

Base is the beauty industry's word for foundation. Make-up artists talk about 'base', meaning the colour, finish and look of a model's skin after they have rendered it flawless and radiant.

BHAs, beta-hydroxy acids, are a popular anti-ageing ingredient – especially during the fruit acid revolution (see pages 218–19). They work in a similar way to AHAs by exfoliating the skin and speeding up cell renewal. A popular BHA is salicylic acid (derived from silver birch bark). BHAs are touted as slightly safer and less aggressive than some fruit acids because the molecules tend to be larger than AHAs and so are less likely to sink deep into the skin and cause irritation. But the bottom line is to treat them with respect and, if you are worried, avoid using them on sensitive skin.

Body sculpting is a term most often used in connection with cellulite-fighting products. Whereas it suggests you can reshape your body, in reality the cream will just enhance the appearance of the skin and possibly improve skin circulation.

Ceramides are rather glamorous scientific-sounding lipids or fats that are found in moisturizers and help prevent moisture loss.

Collagen and elastin are the skin's natural support system. Think of them as rather like the inside of a mattress – with ageing, the 'mattress' naturally becomes weaker. But this weakening process is worsened by smoking and blasting the skin with sunlight, in particular UVA rays. Collagen-protecting and -building creams contain ingredients, such as vitamin C and retinol (see pages 246 and 248), that protect against the natural breakdown of collagen. Putting a 'collagen' cream directly on the skin may not help build collagen within the skin, but it will make the skin feel very smooth.

Demi-matte is a real make-up junkie term. The best action to take with these foundation products is to try them – expect to gain a healthy but not heavily moist finish that is good for oily skin.

Dewy foundations may make you die laughing before buying one because of their ridiculous name, but give the skin a youthful, moist finish rather than a matte one, and are good for dry skins.

Enzymes were the big anti-ageing excitement after AHAs and work in a similar but theoretically less-aggressive way. Rather than using acid to loosen dead skin cells, the right enzymes should not harm living cells but help shift dead, dulling skin cells, leaving the skin fresher and smoother.

Essential oils are pure plant extracts, which are used by aromatherapists trained to know how to dilute and mix the appropriate oil for their clients' needs. You should never apply essential oil directly to the skin.

Humectants attract water from the air to keep the skin nicely moisturized. Common humectants are urea, glycerine and squalene: look for these ingredients in moisturizers.

Keratin is the protein that makes up hair. Layers of overlapping keratin cells look their best when they are lying flat, so that the hair feels smooth and reflects light. Many conditioners and other hair products contain ingredients to help smooth down ruffled keratin to make hair easier to comb and look smoother.

Light-reflecting pigments are often used in concealers and foundations and, as their name suggests, they help refract and bounce light away from the skin. This subtle 'mirror effect' gives the complexion more radiance and makes the skin appear younger. Using a light-reflecting concealer on under-eye circles helps bring light to the darker areas and perks up tired-looking eyes. The pigments are so small that they cannot be detected by the human eye, so there is no danger of looking like a 1970s disco queen.

Liposomes describe a 'delivery system' in which nutrient-filled sacs penetrate deeply into the skin to deliver their contents. Think of them as sophisticated 'skin food' parcels that have the ability to travel deeper into the skin than more straightforward ingredients. They may contain anything from vitamin E to anti-ageing retinol, which can then be released where it is needed in the skin. Nanospheres are similar to liposomes but a more recent invention.

Lymphatic drainage should interest anyone who has a personal crusade against cellulite. Your lymph system is the skin's waste-disposal system. The system becomes sluggish with lack of exercise, swigging toxin-laden drinks or guzzling unhealthy food, and the body's waste disposal is consequently less efficient. By massaging the body along the lymph lines, up towards the heart from the extremities, a sluggish system can be kicked into functioning more efficiently (see also page 17).

Multisticks are foundation sticks that have become popular recently. They tend to give a slightly heavier coverage than most modern foundation formulas, but this is really splitting hairs. A multistick can be carried in your pocket, ready for sneaky retouch moments.

Panthenol (pro-vitamin B5) helps wound-healing and improves moisturization. It is a standard ingredient found in moisturizers.

Photochromatic pigments are the latest ingredients to be included in foundations. Because the pigments have the ability to adjust to different kinds of light and still flatter the skin (unlike older formulas, which were heavier and skin-dulling), you can go from dawn to dusk in a variety of different lights and still look ravishingly natural rather than made-up.

Refining is a beauty term that simply means 'smoothing'.

Retinol is a vitamin A derivative that has been recently launched by cosmetics companies to fight ageing. Retinol is unstable and has to be inserted into delivery systems, such as nanospheres, to control the level in the skin. Retinol creams should be used at night only and a sunscreen worn during the day to protect the slightly more vulnerable skin. Retinol should not be confused with Retin A, Renova or Retinova, which are pharmaceutical drugs and should only be used under medical supervision. Originally used to treat acne patients, these drugs can only be prescribed by doctors and dermatologists.

Sheer coverage is a term used to describe light, almost see-through make-up. A foundation or lipstick offering sheer coverage is the best choice for a natural, subtle look.

Silicone is a common ingredient found in everything from hair products to foundation. It gives silkiness and a 'slip' to formulas. When 'volatile silicones' are included in foundations, they give a smooth application but then evaporate, leaving the pigment 'locked' onto the skin for a more natural, durable finish. In hair products, silicone gives a silky sensation while washing the hair and a shiny, healthy look once it is dry. Hair serums are often silicone-based. Overuse of serum or silicone products can leave hair limp and dirty-looking, but do not despair – just use a 'clarifying' shampoo for a few washes to remove any traces.

Soap-free products are a genuine beauty phenomenon, although a bar of soap-free soap may sound like the Emperor's new clothes. Traditional soap strips the skin's protective acid mantle, leaving it vulnerable to dryness and possibly irritation. Glycerine is a good alternative to traditional soap because it cleans the skin beautifully, comes in bar form and is also a humectant (see page 243) so it will not leave the skin feeling like a piece of chamois leather. If you suffer from eczema or other skin complaints, a soap-free product will help you avoid the skin-drying effects of soap.

Stain is a rather fey way of describing a little bit of colour left on the skin by a lipstick or blusher. I always think the description sounds rather horrid – more like a household washing powder or Lady Macbeth. Think of it as a bonus if you like the natural look, or as a bit of a cop-out if you do not.

Thai massage is a rather end-of-the-millennium form of massage that is gaining in popularity. Think of a combination of yoga and physiotherapy and you are just about there. The therapist will lean on and manipulate your limbs. If you like stretching and have few inhibitions, then you should enjoy this form of massage. Thai massage is not quite as karma sutra as it sounds: it is done with both the therapist and the client fully clothed.

Tightening is a 'beauty speak' term found on many facial and body creams for ageing skins and means that the cream will leave the skin looking firmer, but not necessarily brighter.

Toning, or skin-toning, creams should leave the skin feeling firmer and looking fresher.

Vitamin B as an ingredient is a great moisturizer, but it does not have any more benefit or ability other than that.

Vitamin C is a skin cell health booster, a collagen protector and a radiance improver. A fairly unstable vitamin, it is generally stabilized in an exotic cream or packaging so that it remains potent.

Vitamin E is a good basic moisturizing ingredient that mops up free radicals. Vitamin E will help maintain your skin's healthy balance but it will not have a dramatic effect. Along with other antioxidant vitamins, vitamin E will give the skin a little protection against the damaging effect of ultraviolet rays.

chapter ten

top 20

This is my personal list of luxury and bargain skincare and make-up products. The following products are either suitable for all skin types or are available in different formulas for dry, oily and combination skins.

	Luxury	Bargain
Cleanser	La Prairie Foam Cleanser	Neutrogena Cleansing Bar
Make-up remover	Clinique Take The Day Off	Johnson's Baby Oil
Basic moisturizer	Clarins Multi-Active Day Cream	Vichy Thermal S1 and S2
Night cream	Lancaster Oxygen Repair for Night	A huge helping of your normal daytime moisturizer

Summer moisturizer	Givenchy Natural Glow Protective Skincare	
Eye cream	Estee Lauder Uncircle	Body Shop Elderflower Eye Gel
Emergency balm	Elizabeth Arden Eight Hour Cream	Vaseline Petroleum Jelly
Late night antidote	Guerlain Midnight Secret	
Basic body moisturizer	Clarins Body Firming Cream	E45 Dermatological Cream
Moisturizing face mask	Decleor Hydravital	E45 Dermatological Cream applied thickly
Revitalizing face mask	Clarins Revitalizing Mask	
Eye mask	Decleor Contour des Yeux	
Body smoothers	Clarins Body Firming Cream	Body Shop body brush
Rejuvenating hand cream	Chanel Douceur des Mains	Nivea Original Cream
Foundation	Estée Lauder Futurist	Tesco One Step Make-Up
Concealer	Yves Saint Laurent Touche Eclat	Colourings Lightening Touch
Bronzer	Christian Dior Radiant Touch	
Blusher	Origins Pinch Your Cheeks	Tesco Powder Blush in Rose
Mascara	Yves Saint Laurent Essential Mascara	Boots No 17 Volume Mascara
Fake tan	Estée Lauder Self-Action Super Tan Spray	Body Shop Watermelon Self-Tan Lotion

directory

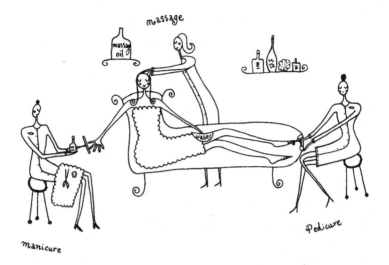

massage

massage oil

manicure

Pedicure

Finding excellent health and beauty experts is often most successfully achieved by word of mouth, so ask your friends or your hairdresser, masseur or beautician for their personal recommendations. There are some areas that are potential charlatan territory, particularly alternative health, and for these it is always advisable to contact a regulating body. The following addresses are a good first 'port of call' and can be relied upon to point you in the right direction, if not help you directly.

**Acne Support
Group**
PO Box 230
Hayes
Middlesex
UB4 9HW
0181 743 2030

**Association of
Chinese Medicine**
78 Haverstock Hill
London
NW3 2BE
0171 284 2898
Call for a list of
practitioners.

**British Association
of Dermatologists**
19 Fitzroy Square
London
W1P 5HQ
0171 383 0266

**The British Wheel
of Yoga**
1 Hamilton Place
Boston Road
Sleaford
Lincolnshire
NG34 7ES
01529 306 851
Call for a list of
qualified yoga
instructors.

The Hale Clinic
7 Park Crescent
London
W1N 2HE
0171 631 0156
Leading holistic
and alternative
health practitioners;
by appointment.

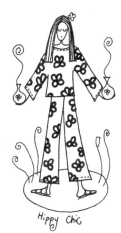

Hippy Chic

**Institute of
Optimum Nutrition**
13 Blade's Court
Deodar Road
London
SW15 2NU
0181 877 9993
Call for nutritional
advice.

Philip Kingsley
54 Green Street
London
W1Y 3RH
0171 629 4004
For hair and scalp
problems.

**Society of
Chiropodists and
Podiatrists**
53 Welbeck Street
London
W1M 7HE
0171 486 3381
Send off for a list
of practitioners.

SALONS AND SPAS

LONDON
Aveda salons:
**The Aveda
Concept Salon
Harvey Nichols**
Knightsbridge
London
SW1X 7XL
0171 201 8610

Regis salons:
Barkers
63 Kensington High
Street
London
W8 5SE
0171 937 5432

Fenwick
63 New Bond Street
London
W1A 3BS
0171 629 3765

Selfridges Spa
5th Floor
400 Oxford Street
London
W1A 1AB
0171 318 3389

Steiner salons:
Steiner Beauty
25A Lowndes Street
London
SW1 9JF
0171 235 3154

**Steiner Hair
& Beauty**
Brent Cross
Shopping Centre
London
NW4 1YP
0181 202 4222

HOME COUNTIES
Regis salons:
Allders
3rd Floor
The Exchange
Shopping Precinct
High Road
Ilford
Essex
IG1 1RR
0181 478 9731

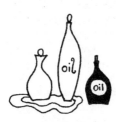

Army & Navy
3rd Floor
Park Street
Camberley
Surrey
GU15 3PG
01276 681446

Army & Navy
4th Floor
105–11 High Street
Guildford
Surrey
GU1 3DU
01483 538598

Army & Navy
1st Floor
St Georges House
Chichester
West Sussex
PO19 1QG
01243 782242

Clements
1st Floor
The Parade
Watford
Hertfordshire
WD1 1LX
01923 238043

Dickins & Jones
1st Floor
28 Acorn Walk
Milton Keynes
Buckinghamshire
MK9 3DJ
01908 607604

Dickins & Jones
3rd Floor
George Street
Richmond
Surrey
TW9 1HA
0181 948 2303

MIDLANDS
Regis salons:
Allders
2nd Floor
The Buttermarket
Centre
Ipswich
IP1 1DU
01473 286455

Beatties
1st Floor
71–80 Victoria Street
Wolverhampton
West Midlands
WV1 3PQ
01902 420409

Denners
2nd Floor
25 High Street
Yeovil
BA20 1RU
01935 444442

Rackhams
6th Floor
35 Temple Row
Birmingham
B2 5JS
0121 236 8806

Rackhams
1st Floor
The Parade
Leamington Spa
Warwickshire
CV32 4DA
01926 339211

Steiner salons:
**Steiner Hair &
Beauty**
25 Corporation
Street
Birmingham
B2 4LF
0121 643 7242

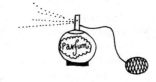

NORTH EAST
Regis salons:
Binns
1st Floor
7 High Row
Darlington
County Durham
DL3 7QE
01325 486876

Binns
3rd Floor
37 Linthorpe Road
Middlesborough
County Durham
TS21 5AD
01642 223157

Binns
226–31 High Street
Lincoln
LN2 1AY
01522 560611

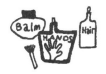

Browns
1st Floor
Daveygate Corner
York
Yorkshire
YO1 2QT
01904 623003

Fenwick
1st Floor
39 Northumberland
Street
Newcastle
NE99 1AR
0191 232 0802

T J Hughes
2nd Floor
High Street
Sheffield
South Yorkshire
S1 1QH
0114 276 9797

Lewis's
Market Street
Manchester
M60 1TX
0161 236 0761

Lewis's
40 Ranelagh Street
Liverpool
L1 1JX
0151 709 8268

NORTH WEST
Regis salons:
Browns
3rd Floor
34–40 Eastgate Row
Chester
CH1 3SB
01244 322965

Kendals
2nd Floor
Deansgate
Manchester
M60 3AU
0161 832 5298

Steiner salons:
**Steiner Hair &
Beauty
Hoopers**
Alderley Road
Wilmslow
Cheshire
SK9 1PB
01652 527469

SOUTH WEST
Regis salons:
Dingles
45–6 Queens Road
Bristol
BS8 1RG
0117 922 5845

WALES
Regis salons:
Howells
14 St Mary's Street
Cardiff
South Glamorgan
CF1 1TT
01222 390645

SCOTLAND
Regis salons:
Jenners
5th Floor
48 Princes Street
Edinburgh
EH2 2YJ
0131 225 9645

Frasers
2nd Floor
21–59 Buchanan
Street
Glasgow
G1 3HR
0141 221 2380

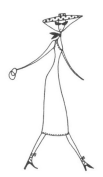

acknowledgements

Some of the best decisions in life are made on whims. Coming up with the idea to write *Faking It!* was one of them. But if it hadn't been for the kindred spirit of Venetia Penfold at Carlton and my brilliant agent Ali Gunn at Curtis Brown, it would never have happened. My biggest thanks go to them for having faith in the idea and turning it into a book.

Other thanks go to my unbelievably supportive and enthusiastic family and friends, who have sniggered encouragingly at the first bits of text and been essential humour-development influences for years. Particular thanks go to Melanie and Nick Purnell, Alex and David Abberton, Camilla Geddes, Tiddy Maitland-Titterton, Hilary Jackson, Ed Averdieck, Charlotte Eagar, Anna Nicholson, Andrew Macdonald, Casilda Grigg, Dan Daley, Harry Ram, Camilla Bashaarat, Mandy Bailey and Miranda Greig. Further huge thanks go to the team at *Woman's Journal* and to Deirdre Vine for her fantastic support and encouragement as an editor. A final thank you to Ann Marie Gardner for encouraging me to develop the original idea.

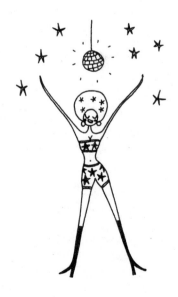